The Bone Biopsy

TOPICS IN BONE AND MINERAL DISORDERS

Series Editor: **Louis V. Avioli, M.D.**
Washington University School of Medicine
St. Louis, Missouri

PAGET'S DISEASE OF BONE
Frederick R. Singer, M.D.

THE BONE BIOPSY
Jenifer Jowsey, D. Phil.

A Continuation Order Plan is available for this series. A continuation order will bring delivery of each new volume immediately upon publication. Volumes are billed only upon actual shipment. For further information please contact the publisher.

The
Bone Biopsy

Jenifer Jowsey, D. Phil.

Mayo Clinic and Mayo Foundation
Rochester, Minnesota

PLENUM MEDICAL BOOK COMPANY
New York and London

Library of Congress Cataloging in Publication Data

Jowsey, Jenifer.
    The bone biopsy.

    (Topics in bone and mineral disorders)
    Bibliography: p.
    Includes index.
    1. Bones — Biopsy. I. Title. II. Series. [DNLM: 1. Bone diseases — Diagnosis.
2. Biopsy — Methods. 3. Bone and bones — Anatomy and histology. WE141 J87b]
RC930.5.J68   616.7'1'0758   77-8647
ISBN 978-1-4684-2381-5

ISBN 978-1-4684-2381-5   ISBN 978-1-4684-2379-2 (eBook)
DOI 10.1007/978-1-4684-2379-2

© 1977 Plenum Publishing Corporation
Softcover reprint of the hardcover 1st edition 1977

227 West 17th Street, New York, N. Y. 10011

Plenum Medical Book Company is an imprint of Plenum Publishing Corporation

To
Fenwick C. Riley, M.D., my husband

Foreword

During the last ten years, the diagnostic approach to disorders of bone and mineral metabolism has benefited considerably from the development of radioimmunoassay and competitive protein-binding techniques for measurements of circulating parathyroid hormone, calcitonin, and biologically active vitamin D metabolites. Accumulated experiences with radiogrametrical and densinometric methods of quantitating appendicular bone mass now facilitate the detection of changes in bone mineral content heretofore unrecognized by routine roentgenographic vertebral analysis.

During this same decade, the diagnosis of metabolic bone disease and the skeletal response to remedial therapeutic maneuvers have also been facilitated by the routine application of the bone biopsy. Improvements in tinctorial techniques, standardization in methodology essential for adequate preparation of thin undecalcified specimens, and the incorporation of tetracycline bone formation or mineralization "markers" should now herald the "routine" use of this diagnostic procedure. Moreover, the compilation and ready availability of reference morphometric data, spanning the prepubescent years characterized by skeletal growth and remodeling and the later senescent period during which bone loss normally proceeds in an unrelenting fashion, allow adequate differentiation between normal age–sex-related changes in skeletal turnover attendant on skeletal maturation and aging and acquired or inherited derangements in bone metabolism.

In this volume, Dr. Jowsey, a renowned international expert in bone metabolism, has presented the case for the bone biopsy. Her vast experience in the analysis of bone morphology and performance of innumerable studies in both experimental animals and human patients continue to enlighten pathologists, orthopedic surgeons, pediatricians, and radiologists, as well as those internists with fundamental interests in the diagnosis and management of metabolic bone disease. This book should prove invaluable to all who appreciate the need for definitive diagnosis of specific disease processes prior to therapeutic intervention.

Louis V. Avioli

St. Louis, Missouri

Preface

Bone is a complex and unusual tissue; complex because it consists of a variety of very differently shaped units linked by joints and ligaments and unusual because of its hardness and the relative paucity of cells. The rigidity of bone depends on the presence of calcium and phosphorus which is embedded in the dense collagen that makes up the bone matrix. The field of bone physiology, therefore, includes many disciplines of science, such as crystallography, endocrinology, and biomechanics. Because the primary function of the skeleton is to store calcium that is made available when inadequate calcium is ingested in the presence of obligatory calcium losses, the relationship between bone metabolism and kidney function, hormone action on bone, kidney, liver, gut, and other target organs and systems must also be part of any discussion of bone as a tissue. No one person can be an expert in all these various disciplines. And perhaps one of the most poorly understood aspects of bone is its morphology.

Bone morphology is a specialized field partly because the hardness of the tissue precludes the use of conventional methods of tissue preparation and staining and also because most of the worthwhile information has come from quantitative evaluation of parameters such as bone mass, volume of unmineralized osteoid, and so forth, rather than qualitative comments. This has necessitated the development of special tools to take the biopsy, special methods for preparing the sections and for evaluating the material. The purpose of this volume is to describe both the special techniques now in use, the information that can be derived from a bone section, and what use this is in the diagnosis of metabolic bone disorders and in understanding the structure and physiology of bone tissue.

Jenifer Jowsey

Rochester, Minnesota

Acknowledgments

I would like to acknowledge, with pleasure, the efforts of my assistants in producing this volume. Mrs. Randi Carlson and Mrs. Joan Toensing have been exceptionally helpful in the preparation of the manuscript; Mrs. C. Yerke, Mr. J. Bronk, Mr. A. Schroeder, Mr. E. Greenwald, and Miss P. Feist have been most industrious and careful in their laboratory work, and Mrs. P. Baker has been of inestimable value in her efforts in recording data and scheduling patient studies. The Medical Illustrations and Photographic Departments, in particular, Mr. Louis Nichols and Miss Jane Hanson, have consistently produced magnificent illustrations which are especially valuable in any morphological treatise. I would also like to thank Dr. M. Coventry and Dr. E. Henderson for their continued encouragement and friendship and also thank my co-workers, Dr. B. L. Riggs and Dr. P. J. Kelly. Research required for a large part of the original data included in this book was supported in part by National Institutes of Health Grant AMO 8658.

Contents

Contents

Chapter 1

Bone Structure

In order to understand adequately the procedures for obtaining
bone biopsies, the methods by which samples are processed,
and most important, the differences which result from different
types of analyses of biopsies, it is necessary to review briefly
the structure of bone tissue.

Bone tissue is formed of a mineralized matrix sparsely in-
terspersed with blood vessels. Because it is mineralized and
therefore hard, the remodeling of the tissue takes place on bone
surfaces by means of two types of cells, the osteoblasts and the
osteoclasts; throughout the bone tissue are osteocytes with pro-
jecting canals which link the blood vascular spaces to each other
and to the endosteal, marrow surface of the bone, producing a
syncytium of fluid-filled channels that allow the transport of
substances throughout the bone tissue.

Bone has been likened to a vascular network lying in a
collagen matrix that is filled with calcium phosphate crystals. A
microopaque injection of radio-dense material gives a clear im-
pression of the vascular supply to bone. In Figure 1, although
there are cross-connections that interconnect the major vessels,
the majority of blood vessels are seen to proceed longitudinally
through cortical bone. Around these vessels are arranged the
Haversian systems, which consist of concentrically organized

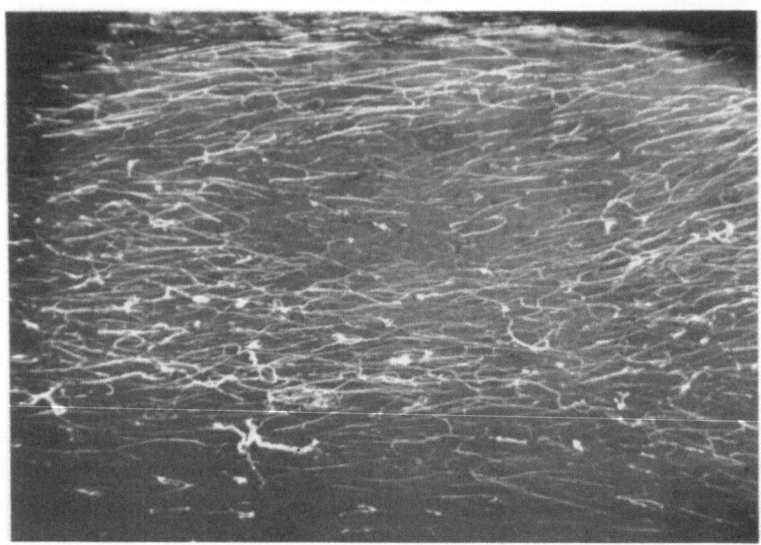

FIGURE 1. Longitudinal section of cortical bone. Microopaque injection demonstrates the vascular network of interconnecting channels running through the bone (magnification ×25).

lamellae of bone bounded by a cement line. The Haversian system is formed by the digging of a tunnel, generally in a longitudinal direction in a long bone, and then the filling in of the tunnel by layers of collagen, which may be compared with sheets of dense connective tissue, and in which the strands are at a slightly different angle from one lamella to another. The alternating lamellae are each approximately 2 μm in width, and, if viewed under polarized light, will produce a birefringent pattern that corresponds to the lamellae of collagen. Because of the circular arrangement of a Haversian system, a Maltese cross will be apparent (Figure 2). In non-Haversian bone, the birefringent pattern will be present if the bone is lamellar, that is, made up of alternating bands of collagen oriented at slightly different angles to each other, but it will not show the Maltese cross. Such lamellar, non-Haversian bone is characteristic of trabecular or spongy bone and of bone laid down on the periosteal and endosteal bone surfaces (Figure 3).

The only type of bone that shows no lamellar pattern is woven bone in which the collagen layers are arranged haphazardly and no pattern can be defined. Woven bone only occurs infrequently and is generally temporary; it is found in the primary spongiosa beneath the epiphyseal plate and also in the new bone of a fracture callus. Although lamellar Haversian bone forms the major part of the skeleton, both lamellar, non-Haversian and, in growing individuals, woven bone occur in the majority of bones of the skeleton.

As bone can be divided into lamellar and nonlamellar, Haversian or non-Haversian, it can also be classified as cortical

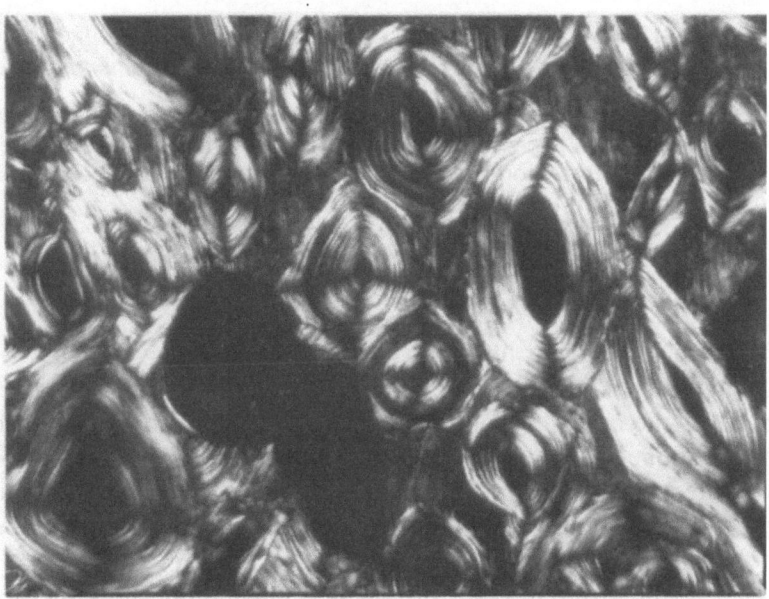

FIGURE 2. Polarized light picture of cortical, secondary Haversian bone. The alternating dark and light bands represent lamellae of collagen of different orientation (magnification × 100).

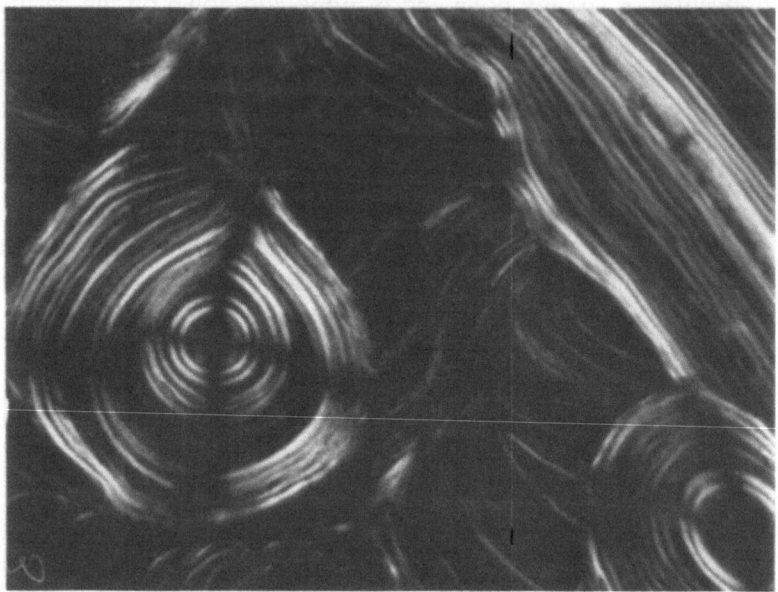

FIGURE 3. Polarized light picture of cortical bone; a well-defined Haversian system is seen on the left surrounded by remains of older Haversian systems. Non-Haversian lamellar bone appears as a band in the upper right (magnification × 250).

or trabecular, types of bone also referred to as compact or spongy bone. The two types are continuous in that the compact bone of the cortex becomes trabecular on the endosteal surface of the bone. The two types differ mainly in their surface-to-volume ratio; this difference results in quantitative variations in the results of analyses of the two types, but not in qualitative differences.

All the different types of bone are made up of the same tissue, which is a collagen-rich matrix containing calcium and phosphate as hydroxyapatite crystals. Cells lie on the bone surface and are scattered sparsely within the tissue.

OSTEOBLASTS AND BONE MATRIX

Bone matrix is synonymous with "osteoid" and refers to the soft part of the bone, which is first deposited by the osteoblasts or can be produced by taking a piece of bone and removing the mineral. It is flexible and rubbery in consistency and is made up largely of lamellae or sheets of collagen with a small amount of glycosaminoglycans (the mucopolysaccharides or ground substances of bone). Osteoid is formed by osteoblasts that secrete small fragments of the collagen fibers and glycosaminoglycans. Osteoblasts are cuboidal cells with a nucleus which generally lies in the cell on the side distant from the bone surface (Figure 4). They form a sheet of cells closely packed

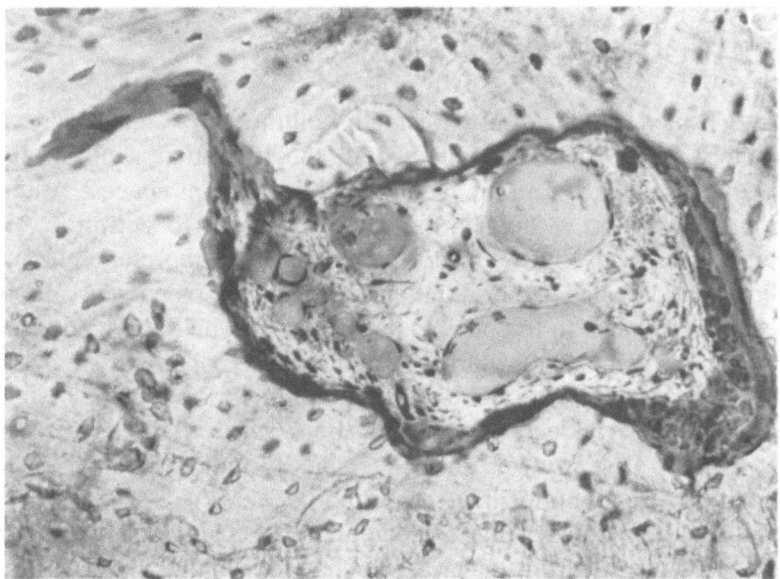

FIGURE 4. A stained, mineralized section of human cortical bone showing a Haversian system where bone formation is just beginning on the right. A thick sheet of osteoblasts is seen, covering a layer of osteoid tissue (magnification × 320).

together on the bone surface and extrude fibrils of collagen and the ground substance of bone. Outside the osteoblast, on the bone side of the cell, the collagen fibrils join lengthwise and three strands spiral round each other while the whole strand spirals in the opposite direction. Such strands pack tightly together with a small percentage of glycosaminoglycans to form the lamellae of bone, the direction of the bands changing approximately every 2 μm. The fibrils become oriented into the orderly arrangement of lamellar bone except in areas where woven, nonlamellar bone is being laid down (Figure 5). Occasionally an osteoblast becomes incorporated into the new matrix as an osteocyte and is connected to the osteoblast layer and to more deeply embedded osteocytes by canaliculi, producing the osteocyte and canalicular system within bone.

OSTEOCYTES AND CANALICULI

Bone contains only a small volume of water (approximately 2%) which is contained in the hydration shell of the hydroxyapatite and in the lacunar and canalicular spaces. An efficient transport system is therefore necessary to permit a metabolic pathway between the living bone and the elements and compounds needed for continued life. The osteocytes lie in elliptical spaces in the bone called lacunae, which are connected to each other by long narrow channels, the canaliculi, that traverse the mineralized bone and eventually exit at the Haversian, endosteal, periosteal, or trabecular bone surface (Figure 6). The canaliculi also connect one Haversian system to another or to adjacent fragments of interstitial bone.

In the lacuna of the osteocyte and the canaliculi there is a layer of unstructured material which separates the cell from the mineralized matrix of the lacuna wall. This material contains a high concentration of glycosaminoglycans and occasionally collagen fibrils. The osteocyte cell wall may be smooth and may lie close to the lacunar wall. Such osteocytes are in the forming

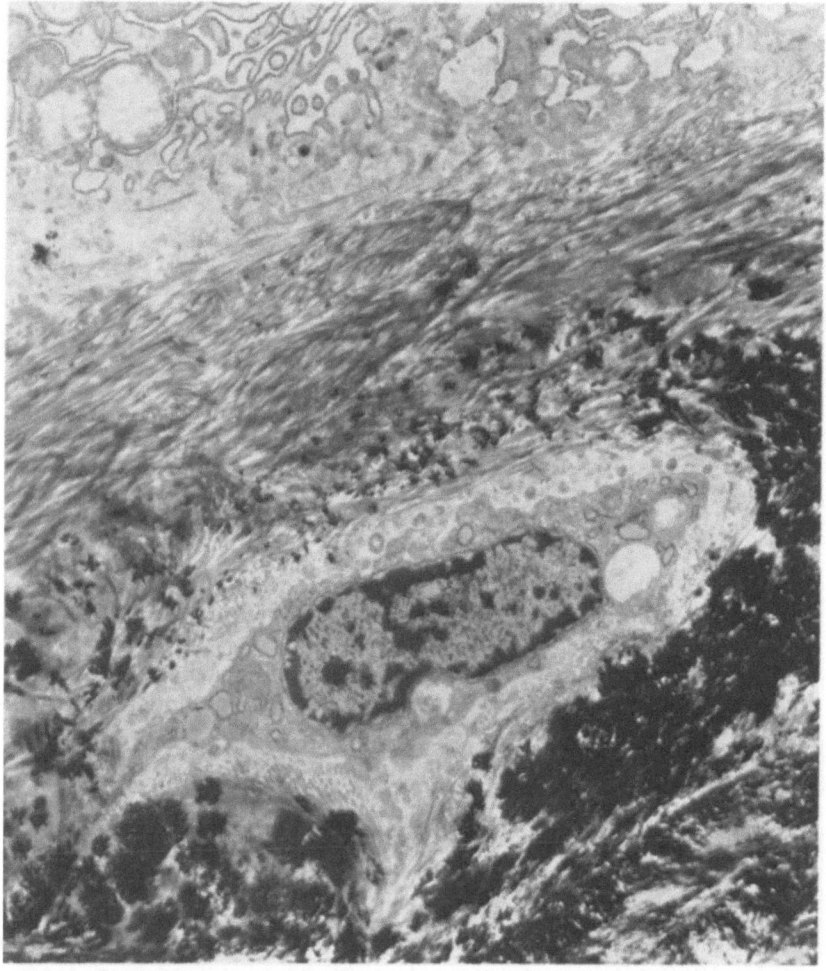

FIGURE 5. Electron microscope appearance of an osteoblast laying down collagen fibrils. An osteoblast has become embedded in the collagen and demonstrates the lacunar and canalicular structure characteristic of an osteocyte. The mineralization front appears as a scattering of dense granules in the area of new collagen (magnification about ×10,000) (courtesy of J. A. Maynard, Ph.D.).

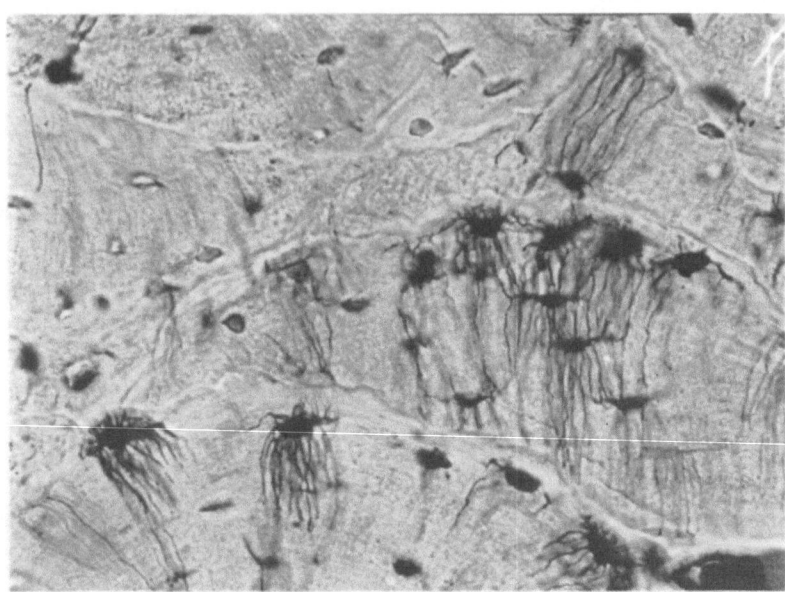

FIGURE 6. Unstained section of human cortical bone. The bone is mineralized and some osteocytes and canaliculi are filled with air and appear black. The intricate connection between osteocytes can be seen; canaliculi can be seen to cross the cement lines which form the boundary of each fragment of interstitial bone (magnification × 500).

phase, and the cytoplasm contains a distinct endoplasmic reticulum (Figure 7). There are a nucleus, a Golgi apparatus, and dense mitochondria also within the cytoplasm of the osteoblastic or formative osteocyte (Baud and Dupont, 1962; Remagen *et al.*, 1969). The resting or inactive osteocytes, sometimes referred to as degenerative osteocytes, have a wider border of material between the cell wall and the lacunar wall, and vacuoles appear in the cytoplasm and mitochondria (Figure 8). Flocculent material is often present in the pericellular space (Jande, 1971).

Osteocytes are also capable of bone resorption. In this phase there are few mitochondria, while the Golgi apparatus is

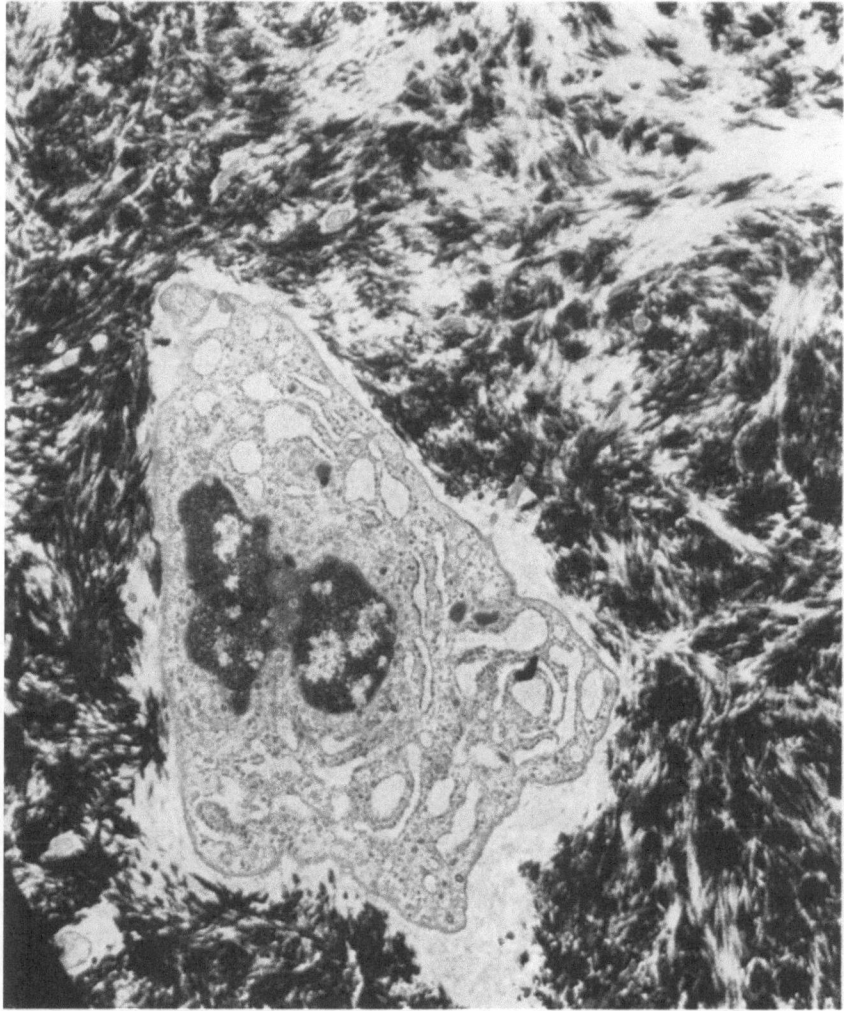

FIGURE 7. Electron micrograph showing a young formative osteocyte in a lacuna in mineralized bone. Small circular holes in the matrix are the canaliculi cut in cross section containing a projection of the osteocyte (magnification about × 10,000) (courtesy of J. A. Maynard, Ph.D.).

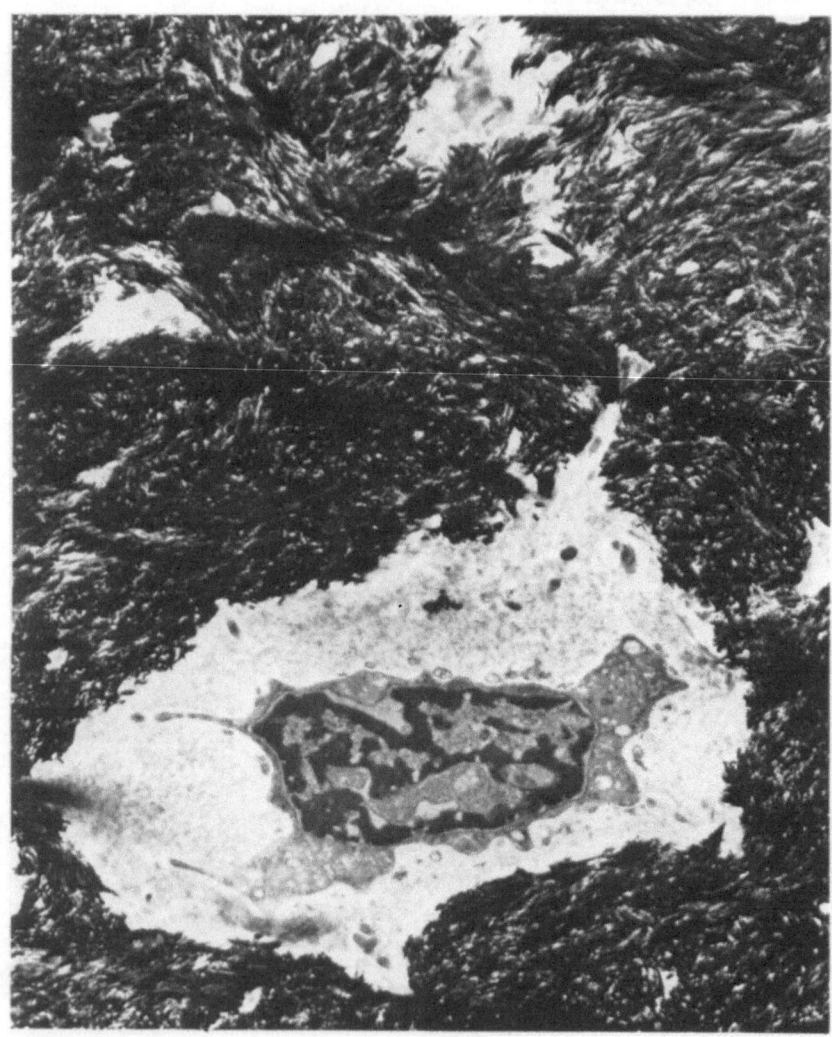

FIGURE 8. Electron micrograph of a mature, inactive or degenerative osteocyte in mineralized bone (magnification about × 10,000) (courtesy of J. A. Maynard, Ph.D.).

large and associated with prominent vesicles (Jande, 1971). There may be lysosomes in the cytoplasm and flocculent material may be present in the perilacunar space. The presence of the lysosomes and the apparent increase in lacunar size found around such osteocytes have suggested that there is destruction of bone occurring (Jande and Bélanger, 1973). It must be emphasized that the presence of large osteocytes alone is not suf-

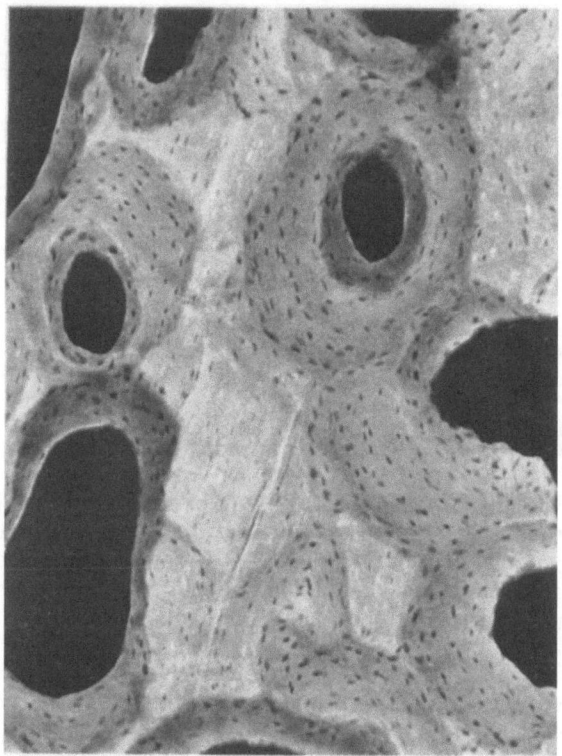

FIGURE 9a. Microradiograph of a cross section of human cortical bone showing osteocyte lacunae in Haversian and interstitial, lamellar bone. Some osteocyte lacunae are partially or completely filled with hydroxyapatite, indicating necrosis and absence of the osteocyte (magnification × 100). From Jowsey, 1973a.

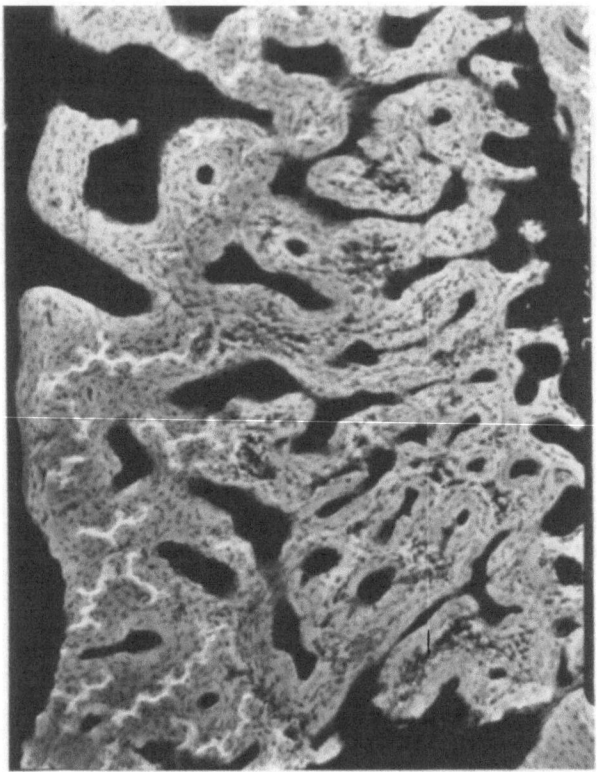

FIGURE 9b. Microradiograph of a cross section of cortical rabbit bone. Large osteocyte lacunae are normally present in the woven bone between the primary Haversian systems. The white irregular lines on the left are struts of mineralized cartilage that have not been remodeled (magnification × 100).

ficient evidence for resorption by osteocytes or osteocytic osteolysis; woven bone is formed with large irregular osteocytes that are somewhat less elliptical and more dense than the regular osteocyte lacunae of lamellar bone (Baud and Auil, 1971). If bone resorption occurs around an osteocyte, it is generally in response to increased levels of circulating parathyroid hormone and the cells thus affected are generally randomly spaced throughout the bone and not associated with woven bone (Figures 9a–f).

The canaliculi that connect the lacunae to each other contain projections of the osteocyte that travel along the canaliculus and meet projections from neighboring osteocytes. These projections abut onto each other and form a tight junction, presumably allowing physiological as well as anatomical continuity between adjacent osteocytes. The canaliculi are most frequently

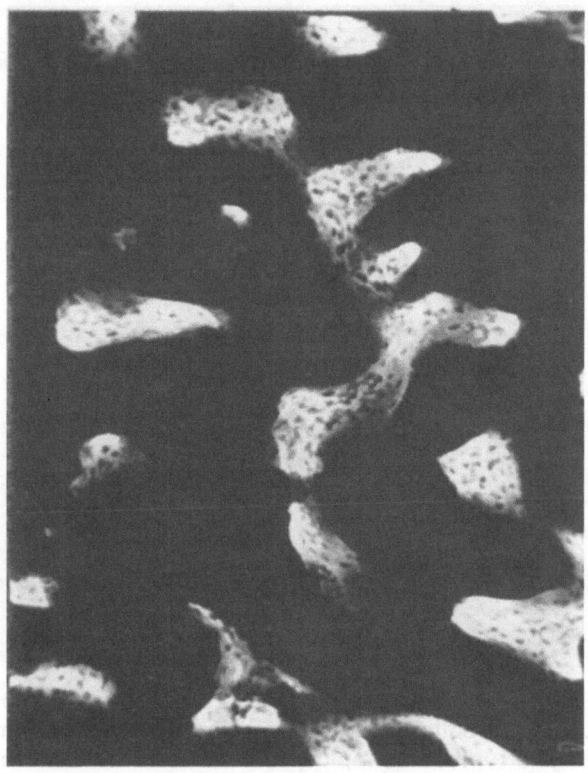

FIGURE 9c. Microradiograph of metaplastic bone trabeculae from a patient with primary hyperparathyroidism. The osteocytes are large and irregular (magnification × 100). From Riggs *et al.*, 1965.

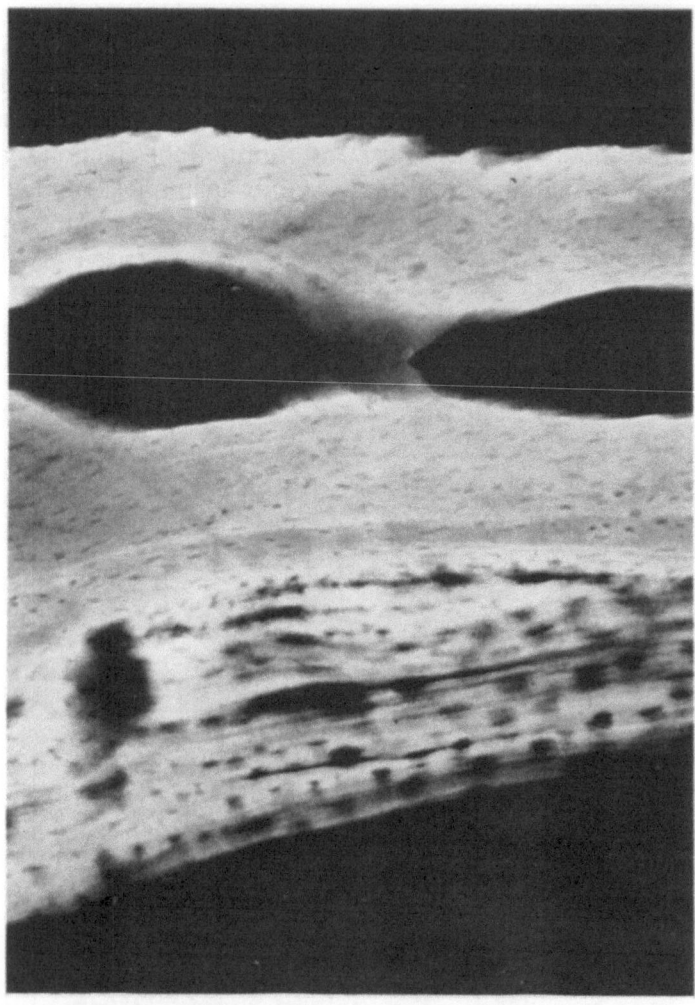

FIGURE 9d. Microradiograph of a cross section of cortical bone from a human being given sodium fluoride and calcium. The endosteal bone represents rapidly formed new bone that contains osteocyte lacunae that are surrounded by poorly mineralized bone (magnification × 100).

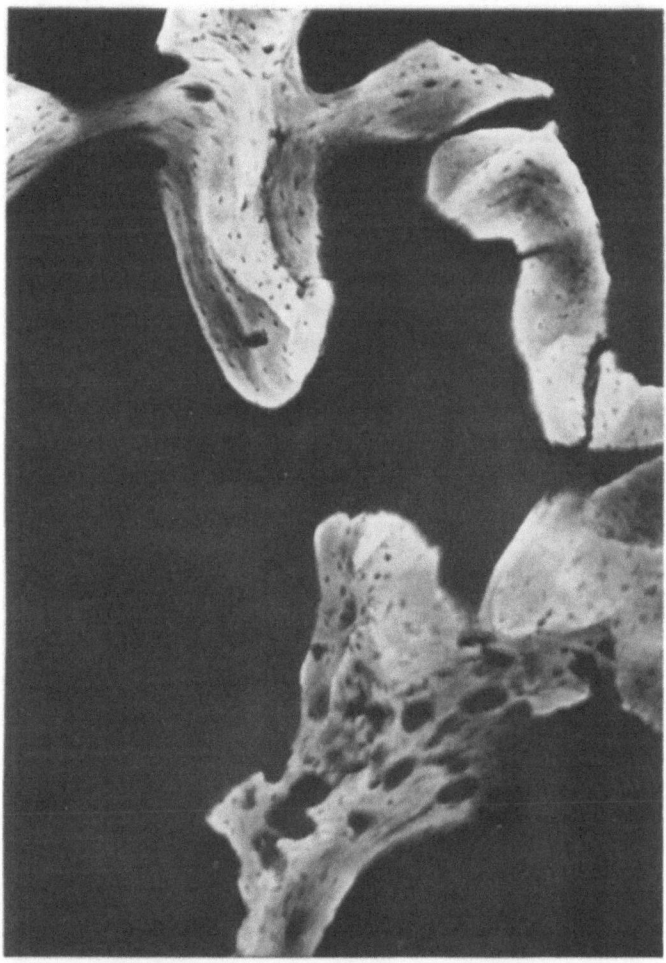

FIGURE 9e. Microradiograph of trabecular bone from a patient with hyperparathyroidism showing osteocytic osteolysis that has occurred in some areas of previously normal bone. Both matrix and mineral have been removed in the process of resorption by the osteocyte (magnification × 100).

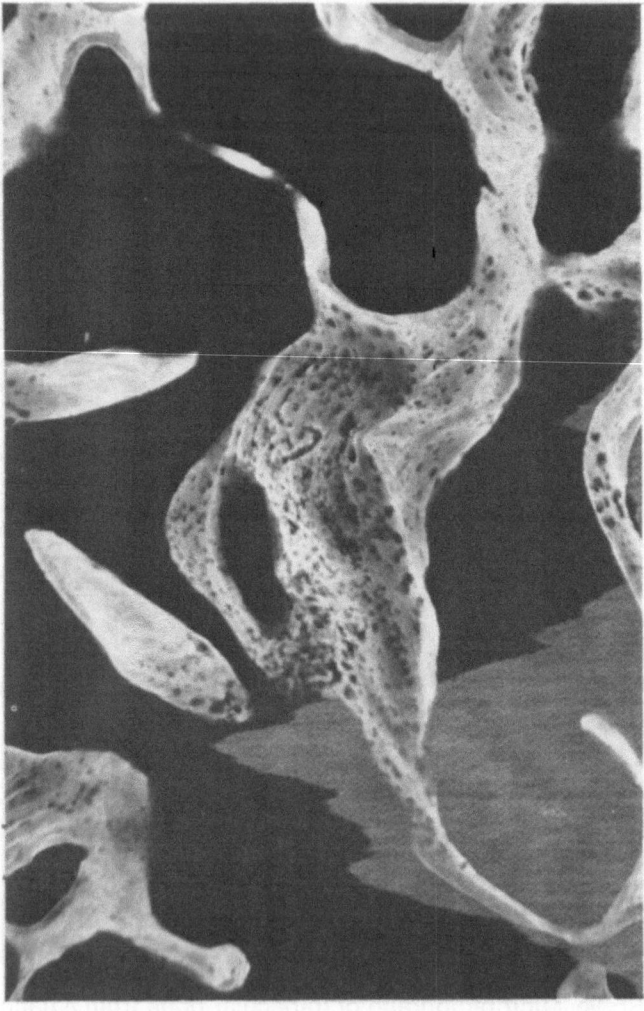

FIGURE 9f. Microradiograph of trabecular bone from a patient with Mast cell disease. The osteocytes are more uniformly affected than in hyperparathyroidism (magnification × 100).

unbranched and of small diameter, exiting singly from the lacunar wall. However, occasional canaliculi of larger diameter branch almost immediately on leaving the lacuna, each branch containing a projection of the osteocyte (Pawlicki, 1975). Such canaliculi occur almost invariably at the apex of the lacuna.

The primary function of the osteocyte and canalicular system is one of transport. Through the pericellular space nutrients and metabolic products pass from the blood to the bone and efficiently maintain the life of the bone and the continued exchange between elements in the blood and in the bone mineral. It has been suggested that bone cannot exist without becoming necrotic unless it is within a millimeter of a vascular channel; that this is not so is evident from the large areas of bone with no vascular supply that remain viable. Such bone is deposited in the process of lamellar, non-Haversian bone formation and is frequently found in the long bones of animals, where secondary Haversian remodeling is often less evident than in the bone of human beings of a similar skeletal maturity (Figure 10).

BONE MINERALIZATION

After the osteoblasts become embedded in the matrix to form osteocytes, the matrix becomes mineralized. Bone mineral consists of hydroxyapatite crystals which are of calcium, phosphorus, hydroxyl ions, and trace elements arranged in a regular fashion to form the crystal lattice. The mineralization of unmineralized osteoid takes place at the mineralization front, which is a narrow band, about 2 to 3 μm in width, that separates the osteoid border from the mineralized bone. In the light microscope it appears as a granular band of slightly dark material in an undemineralized section. If mineralization is delayed, the mineralization front is broadened and may be patchy (Figure 11). In the electron microscope the mineralization front is seen to be a number of small foci of crystals (Figure 5).

Mineralization of bone appears to be initiated inside matrix

vesicles that are found in the extracellular matrix. It is not yet
clear whether the matrix vesicles originate from mitochondrial
granules or are formed *de novo* in the extracellular matrix (Howell, 1976). After the formation of dense aggregates of calcium
and phosphorus within the vesicle membrane, larger hydroxyapatite crystals can be seen, which burst through the membrane
and eventually become mature crystals. This process occurs
very rapidly, approximately 75% of the full degree of bone
mineralization, or a width of approximately 1 μm, occurring in
24 h. The remainder of the mineral is deposited in an ever-
decreasing rate until mineralization is complete (Figure 12). The
completion of mineralization generally occurs from the inner

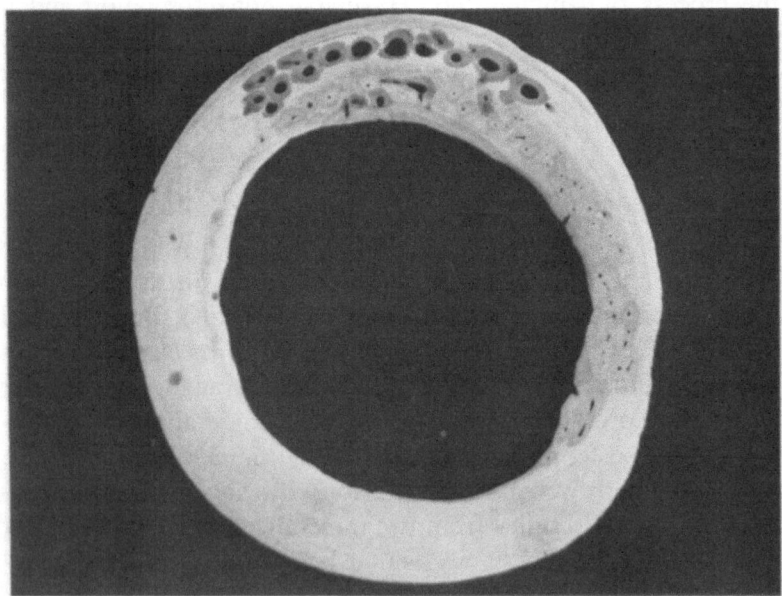

FIGURE 10. Microradiograph of a cross section of cortical bone
from a monkey. Some secondary Haversian remodeling has occurred in one area. The majority of bone consists of lamellar non-
Haversian bone without vascular channels (magnification × 15).

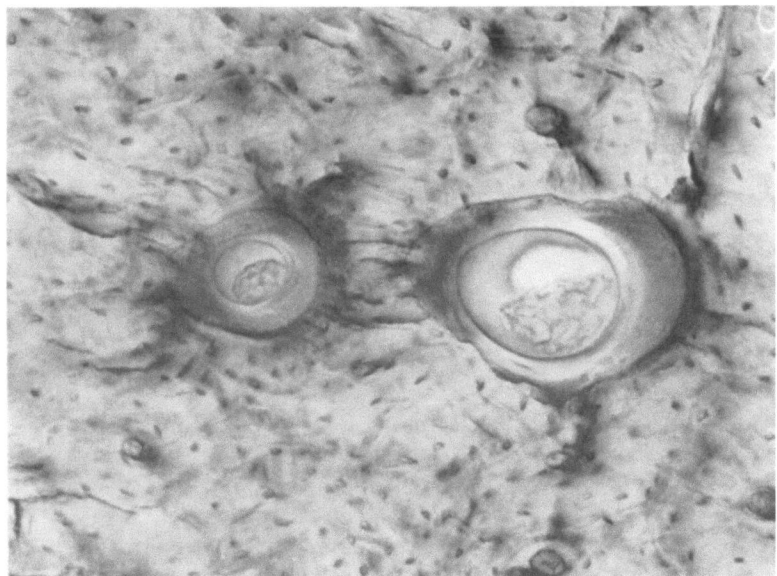

FIGURE 11. An unstained, mineralized section of cortical bone from an animal given EHDP, a diphosphonate. The mineralization front is wide and is not found uniformly around the whole osteoid border in the Haversian system on the right (magnification × 250). From: Jowsey *et al.*, 1970.

vascular surface of the Haversian system, or from the marrow side of the trabeculum, inward toward the cement line. The result is that as soon as bone formation ceases, the bone surface appears hypermineralized in relation to the bone behind it.

OSTEOCLASTS

In contrast to the osteoblast, the osteoclast is generally multinucleate, and it is larger. Rather than occurring in sheets on the bone surface, osteoclasts are found singly in indentations, the Howship's lacunae, that they have produced by ero-

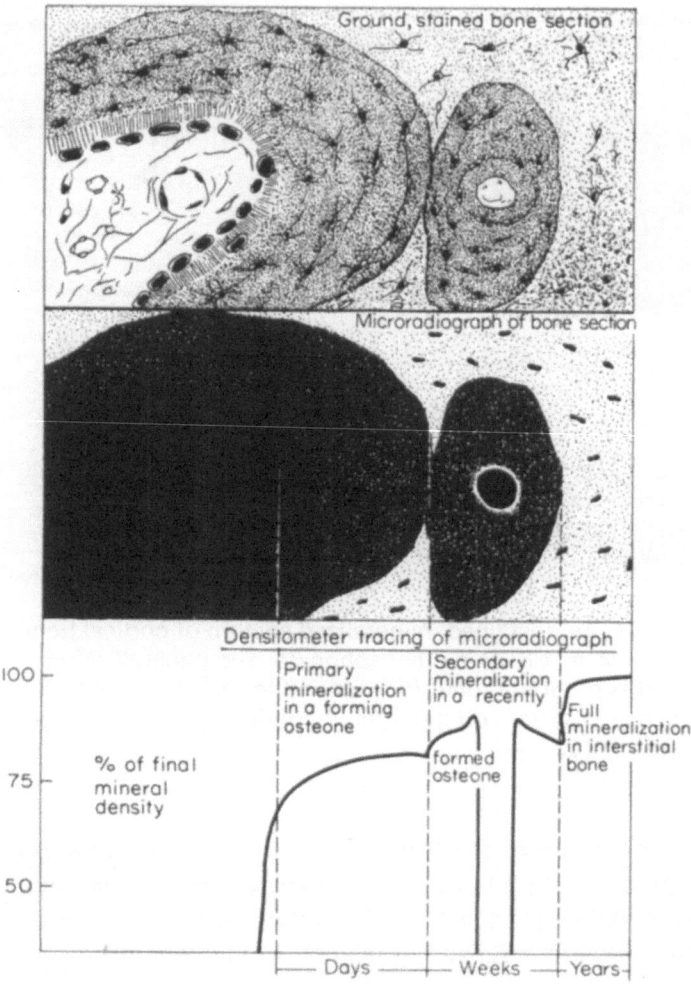

FIGURE 12. Diagram of the process of mineralization in new bone.

sion of mineralized bone (Figure 13). The nuclei may number from 1 to 200, the number depending on the size of the cell and, in thin sections, on the plane of section of the preparation. An active osteoclast lies close to a mineralized bone surface, and the nuclei are found on the side of the cell away from the bone.

On the side of the cell adjacent to the bone is the brush border (or ruffled border) which consists of many villi that protrude from the cell and interdigitate with the mineralized bone surface (Figure 14). The presence of a ruffled border is essential for the proper resorptive function of the cell. If the ruffled border is absent, as in osteopetrosis, no bone resorption takes place, although the bone is filled with osteoclasts. The osteoclasts produce lysosomal enzymes such as acid phosphatase, and both malic and lactic dehydrogenase (Walker, 1972). There are also high concentrations of citrate in osteoclasts, which is involved in the mobilization of calcium from the bone.

Osteoclasts resorb bone by destroying both the collagen and the bone mineral. Electron microscopy reveals hydroxyapatite crystals and collagen fibers within the cell in vacuoles that project down into the cell cytoplasm and that give the cell the foamy appearance which is characteristic of an active osteoclast. Within the cell the collagen and crystals are further degenerated to hydroxyproline, calcium and phosphorus, which are released into the extracellular fluid and the blood. The process of resorption has been termed endocytosis, and morphological evidence, again from electron microscopic studies, has shown that the collagen and mineral are removed at essentially the same time (Lucht, 1972; Bonucci, 1974). The initial stage of resorption is extracellular and results in fragmentation of the mineralized bone. The fragments are phagocytosed by the osteoclast and the pieces are digested intracellularly. It is possible that the first component of bone to be disassociated is the glycosaminoglycan portion of the matrix, which permits the detachment of the crystals from the collagen and the initial step in collagen fibril breakdown. The intracellular digestion takes place mainly in the lysosomal vacuoles of the osteoclast.

Osteoclasts are on the average six times as large as osteoblasts and have six times as many nuclei (Owen, 1971). As indicated by experimental studies, the activity per unit surface of bone of osteoclasts is also greater than that of osteoblasts. Therefore, although there is obviously a great variation in the resorptive activity of different cells, the osteoclast appears to be

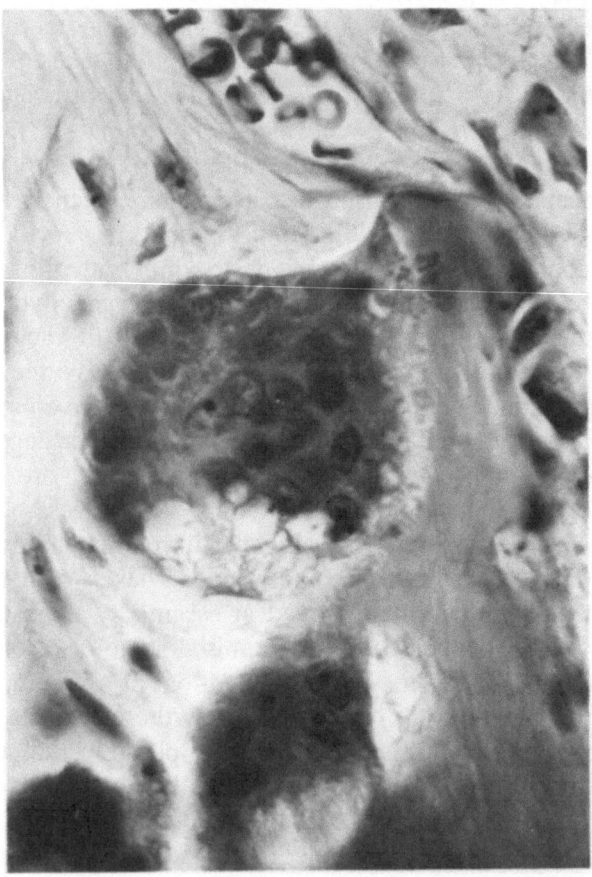

FIGURE 13. Stained histological preparation of an osteoclast. The cell is multinucleate and contains vacuoles; a brush border lies between the cell and the mineralized bone (magnification × 600) (courtesy of Mr. B. Boothroyd).

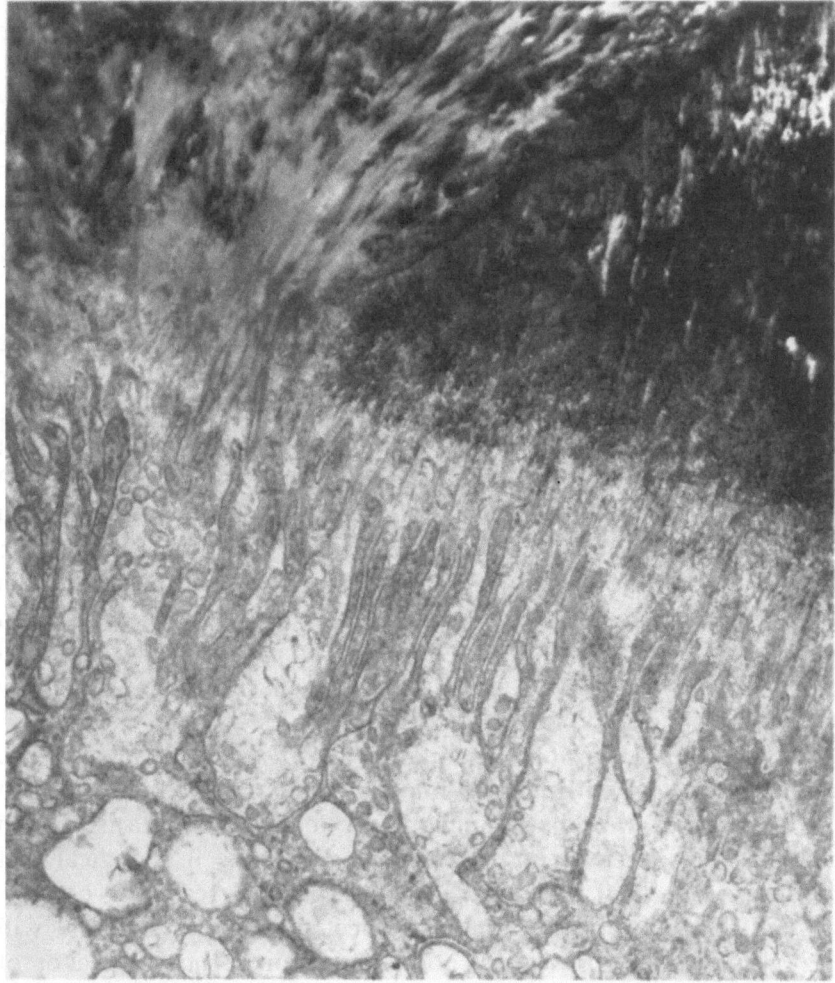

FIGURE 14. Electron micrograph of an osteoclast, showing part of the ruffled or brush border lying on the mineralized bone surface. The brush border is made up of many villi with vacuoles between and behind them, in which hydroxyapatite crystals can be seen (magnification about ×20,000) (courtesy of J. A. Maynard, Ph.D.).

able to destroy bone more efficiently than osteoblasts can form it.

Although the vast majority of bone resorption takes place as a result of osteoclastic activity, cells other than typical osteoclasts can be found in Howship's lacunae and are seen in significant numbers in bone-losing diseases, suggesting their role as mediators of bone destruction. Mononuclear osteoclasts can obviously be produced in a section as the result of sectioning artifact, when the tip of a cell is cut off and lies against the bone surface of the section. However, genuine mononuclear osteoclasts have been observed in bone resorption areas (Figure 15) (Ch'uan, 1931; Tonna, 1960). In multiple myeloma the myeloma cells of the marrow appear to be responsible for bone loss; they are adjacent to the bone surface and in many instances of myeloma characterized by rapid bone loss, osteoclasts are not prolific. Recently Mundy and co-workers (Mundy *et al.*, 1974) have suggested that the myeloma cells produce a substance that stimulates osteoclasts to resorb bone, their studies relying largely on the appearance of osteoclasts in bone biopsies from patients with multiple myeloma. Nevertheless, bone destruction appears to occur in areas where osteoclasts are not present and frequently enough to make it possible that myeloma cells may cause bone resorption directly.

Osteoclasts possess the ability to resorb mineralized bone and also to distinguish the mineral content of the bone adjacent to them. Since their function is calcium homeostasis, which they achieve by resorbing mineralized bone, it is logical that these cells will not achieve their purpose by resorbing osteoid. Osteoclasts show a great reluctance to resorb osteoid and will also discriminate against poorly mineralized bone in favor of fully mineralized bone. If bone is covered by osteoid tissue, osteoclasts can be seen to penetrate the osteoid and resorb the mineralized bone behind (Figure 16). The phenomenon has been termed "dissecting resorption" because the appearance is one of mineralized bone that has been split by a wedge or cone of resorption, and the space filled with connective tissue (Figure 17).

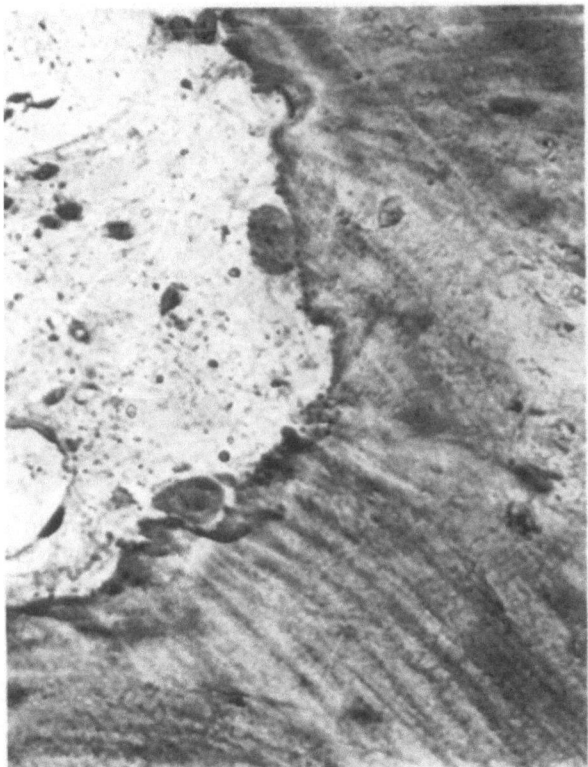

FIGURE 15. A stained, mineralized bone section demonstrating small mononuclear cells in Howship's lacunae that appear to be resorbing bone (magnification ×640).

The presence of fibrous connective tissue in the past has been taken as an indication of increased resorption, to the point at which "osteitis fibrosa" was synonymous with above-normal levels of bone resorption. In advanced primary hyper-parathyroidism, the increased bone resorption was frequently associated with the presence of fibrous connective tissue. The more recent basis of diagnosis of hyperparathyroidism on elevated serum calcium levels or on increased immunoreactive

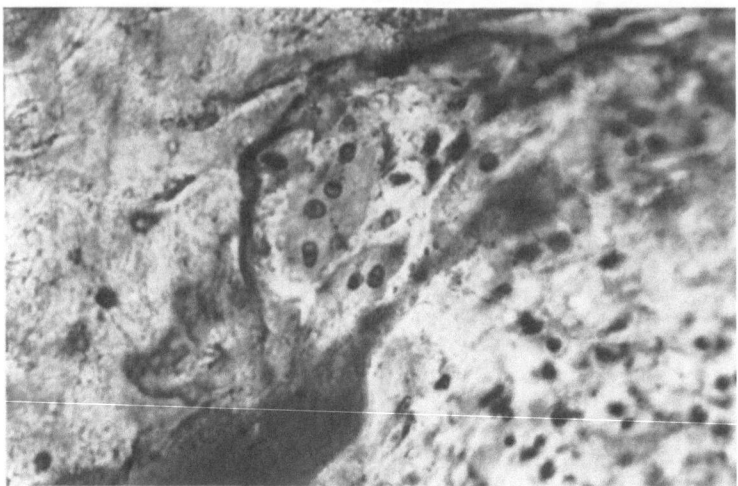

FIGURE 16. Stained, mineralized section of bone from a patient with secondary hyperparathyroidism due to renal failure. Osteoclasts have burrowed through the darkly stained osteoid and are resorbing the mineralized bone behind (magnification × 520).

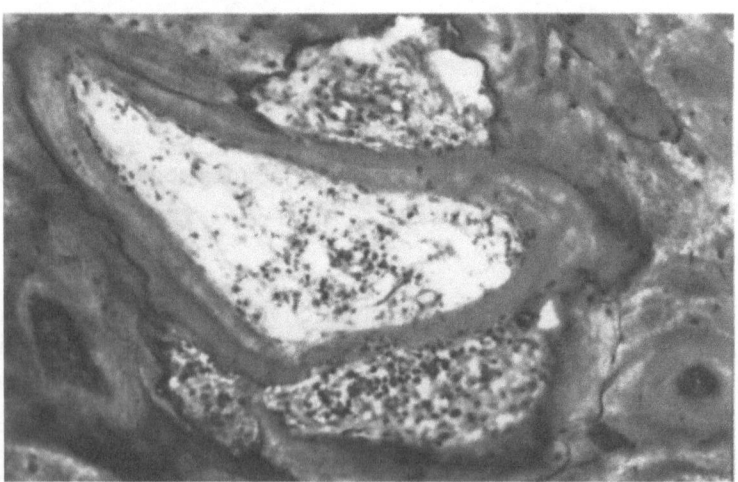

FIGURE 17. Stained, mineralized section of bone from a patient with renal osteodystrophy. Two resorption cavities lie behind the osteoid border (magnification × 450).

parathyroid hormone levels has made it less likely that the bone disease has progressed to the point of osteitis fibrosa. The latter appears to be an expression of excessive parathyroid hormone stimulation.

When bone resorption stops, a border of high mineral density appears on the old resorption surface. A cement line is formed as new bone is deposited and represents the line of demarcation between a zone of resorption and new bone formation. It is histologically identifiable as a narrow line with a high concentration of glycosaminoglycans and calcium, which is relatively poor in collagen (Figure 18). It is somewhat less than 1 μm in thickness and therefore can rarely be seen on a microra-

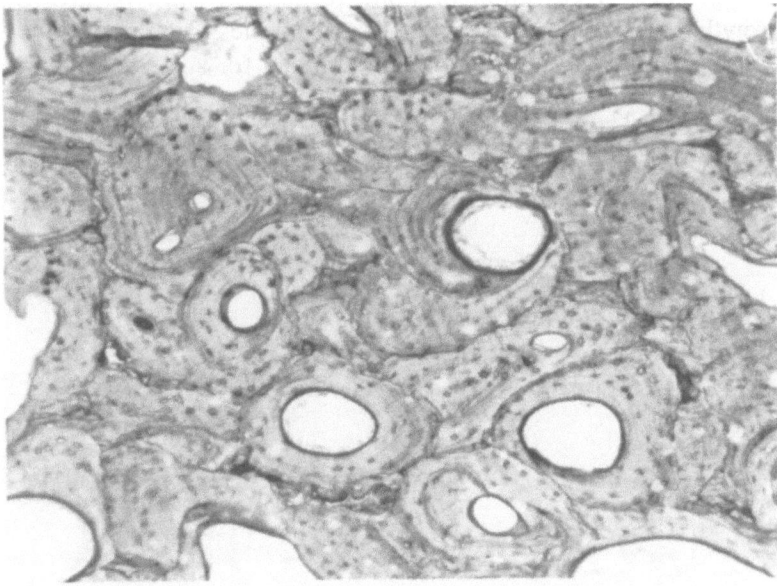

FIGURE 18. A stained, mineralized section of cortical, human bone containing many secondary Haversian systems. Each Haversian system is surrounded by a thin, dark line, the cement line. Within each osteone there are less distinct darker zones, which represent collagen fibers that are differentially stained (magnification × 125).

diograph. A cement line forms the boundary of a Haversian system or of a band of non-Haversian lamellar bone. Remains of Haversian systems, formed as continued resorption and formation in cortical bone replace previously formed Haversian systems, will also be surrounded by cement lines. Such fragments of old Haversian systems will constitute the interstitial lamellae and differ from complete Haversian systems in that they do not contain a central Haversian canal.

If bone formation ceases, a layer similar to a cement line is laid down, which appears as a glucosaminoglycan-rich line within a Haversian system or a band of lamellae in a trabeculum. Such a structure is called a line of arrested growth and in contrast to a cement line, it does not represent an area where resorption ceased and formation started. Since immobilization will produce a cessation of bone formation, lines of arrested growth are frequently seen in bone samples from individuals who have been at bed rest or immobilized for some reason.

Chapter 2

Cell Origins

It is obvious from morphological studies that osteocytes originate from osteoblasts. However, the origin of osteoblasts and osteoclasts have been subject to controversy. Until recently, original investigations by Young (1962) and Tonna (1965) had suggested that osteoblasts and osteoclasts both originate from mesenchyme or progenitor cells; these cells are independently stimulated by different hormones or different stresses and differentiate into osteoclasts and osteoblasts, which resorb and form bone, respectively. There is some evidence that osteoclasts may form from osteogenic cells (Tonna and Cronkite, 1968). However, the studies were carried out in young growing rats and may represent the rapid change from bone formation to bone resorption in bone that is in the process of rapid turnover. The same situation may exist for infants, but it is not likely to be true of the bone of juveniles or adults of the human species. Nevertheless, it represents a rapid cycling of nuclear material that occurs at a slower rate in all bone cells. The origin of osteoclasts from osteoblasts has been challenged by Young (1964). This investigator rightly points out that osteoblasts which coalesce to form an "osteoclast" will still have the properties and the enzyme system of an osteoblast and will therefore merely be a multinucleate osteoblast. Young also provides ample evidence for the existence of progenitor cells which are the source of both the osteoblast and the osteoclast. Later work has confirmed the independent origin of osteoclasts and osteoblasts from undifferentiated progenitor cells. Frost's concept of the "cytodynamic" sequence of events in bone remodeling is that a mesenchymal cell is transformed or modulated into an osteoclast which resorbs bone; when the stimulus for resorption ceases, the osteoclast is despecialized into a mesenchyme cell and later progenitor cells differentiate into osteoblasts if there is stimulus for bone formation (Villanueva, 1973). In cortical bone where rapid bone turnover is occurring, the sequence very frequently proceeds with no inactive period and little lapse of time between them. This can be illustrated in a stained section where osteoclastic resorption is taking place in a Haversian system followed, at a short interval, by bone formation. The interval between resorption and formation activity, observed in longitudinal sections in the dog, is approximately 300 μm (Jaworski and Lok, 1976). In this interval osteoclasts dedifferentiate into progenitor cells before being restimulated to form osteoblasts. In adult man, osteoclastic bone resorption occurs and leaves an inactive surface that may exist for a long time. Indeed, inactive Haversian systems and trabecular surfaces where resorption of bone was the last cellular event are found approximately nine times more frequently than resorption or forming spaces, and they contain fibroblasts and blood vascular elements only.

The origin of osteoclasts and osteoblasts was most recently considered by Rasmussen and Bordier. On the basis of scanty evidence purporting to show osteoclasts breaking up into osteoblasts, these authors suggested that osteoblasts were derived from osteoclasts (Rasmussen and Bordier, 1973). However, the morphological appearance to support this claim has not been substantiated by any other investigators, and the data of Owen (1971), which were erroneously used to support their theory, in fact suggest a separate cell origin for the osteoclast and osteoblast. Tritiated thymidine incorporation *in vivo* is first seen in progenitor cells, which are referred to as preosteoblasts and preosteoclasts; after a period of 48 h the tritium label appears in both osteoclasts and osteoblasts at the same time (Young, 1962; Owen, 1971). If osteoblasts were derived from osteoclasts, the label would have appeared sooner in the osteoclasts.

More sophisticated studies have indicated a separate origin of the osteoclast and osteoblast. Parabiotic union between two rats allows transfer of only the blood cell elements between the two animals. If one animal is injected with tritiated thymidine as a nuclear label in order to mark the bone cells, and cell proliferation is discouraged in the second by irradiation, only the osteoclasts appear labeled in the second animal (Gothlin and Ericsson, 1973). This study not only showed that osteoblasts and osteoclasts are derived from separate cell origins, but also that the osteoclast is derived from a hematogenic cell, while the osteoblast is derived from a fibroblast type of progenitor cell. Later studies by Buring (1975) confirmed that blood-borne cells form the osteoclasts, while osteoblasts are derived from perivascular mesenchymal cells (Figure 19). Using a chimera com-

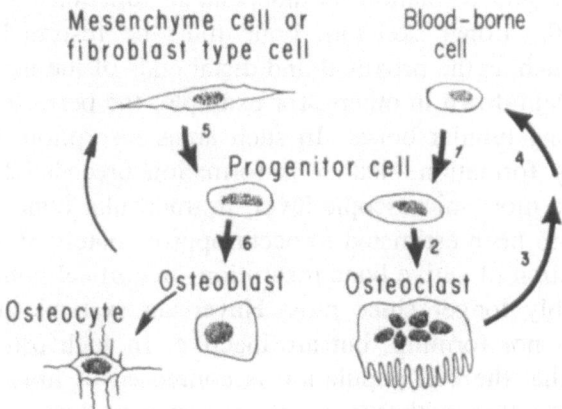

FIGURE 19. Diagram illustrating bone cell dynamics, showing the separate cell origins of osteoclasts and osteoblasts and the formation of an osteocyte from an osteoblast.

posed of Japanese quail limb tissue grown in a chicken embryo membrane system, Kahn also demonstrated the separate cell origins of the osteoblast and osteoclast (Kahn and Simmons, 1975) (Figure 20).

The experimental evidence, therefore, overwhelmingly supports the concept that the two cells responsible for bone turnover, the osteoblast and the osteoclast, originate from different precursor cells. The mesenchymal, osteoprogenitor or progenitor cell is a small fibroblast-like cell found adjacent to areas where resorption and formation are taking place, and it differentiates into an osteoblast (Figure 21). On the other hand, osteoclasts are derived from hematogenous cells and do not form osteoblasts, nor are the two cells linked in their activity or origin. From the theoretical standpoint, it would not serve the purpose of the skeleton, either in its role as a source of calcium or as an intricately designed supporting structure, to require bone formation to be the inevitable consequence of resorption either temporarily or geographically. The remodeling of bones that takes place to give the skeleton its final adult form and the turnover of bone that continues throughout life both demand that resorption and formation be independent functions. In order to form a functional skeleton, bone must be resorbed in some places, such as the proximal and distal ends of the marrow cavity, and laid down in others, for example, the periosteal surface of the long tubular bones. In such areas resorption is not followed by formation, neither is formation preceded by resorption. At a more microscopic level, in trabecular bone, bone formation has been estimated to occur approximately 36 days after the cessation of active bone resorption. In cortical bone the time is probably longer since most Haversian systems are neither resorbing nor forming, but are inactive. In such osteones it is evident that the cell population is composed of fibroblasts and cells associated with the vascular systems; there are no osteoclasts waiting to become osteoblasts (Parfitt, 1973). In order to maintain a normal serum calcium level bone is constantly remodeled in the adult, and this bone turnover represents the constant need for an available supply of calcium, which is

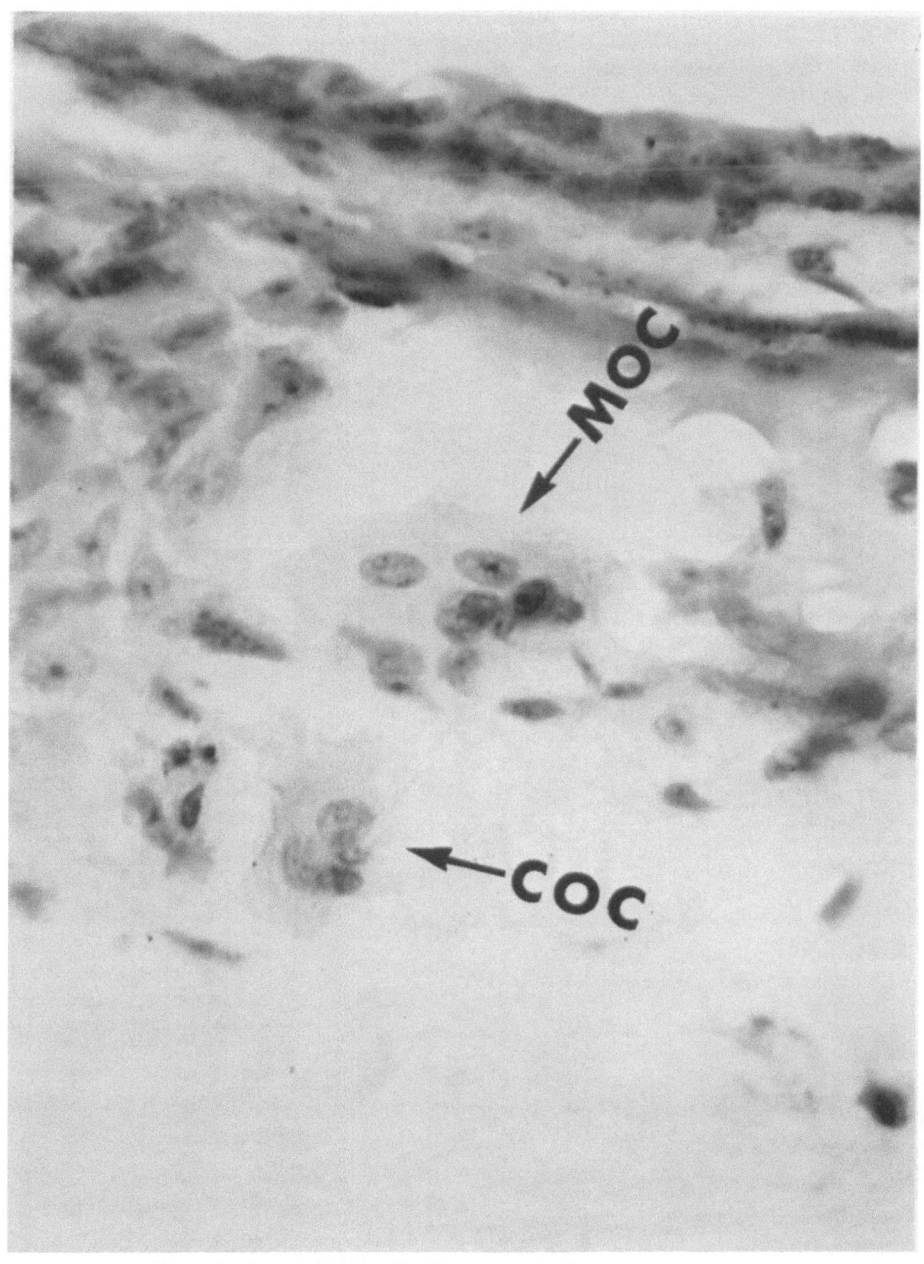

FIGURE 20. Two osteoclasts in a tissue culture preparation of a quail rudiment that has been grown on the chorioallantoic membrane of a chick embryo for 8 days. One osteoclast (COC) contains nuclei of the chick type while the other (MOC) possesses nuclei of both quail and chick (Feulgen stain; magnification × 1250) (courtesy of A. J. Kahn, Ph.D.).

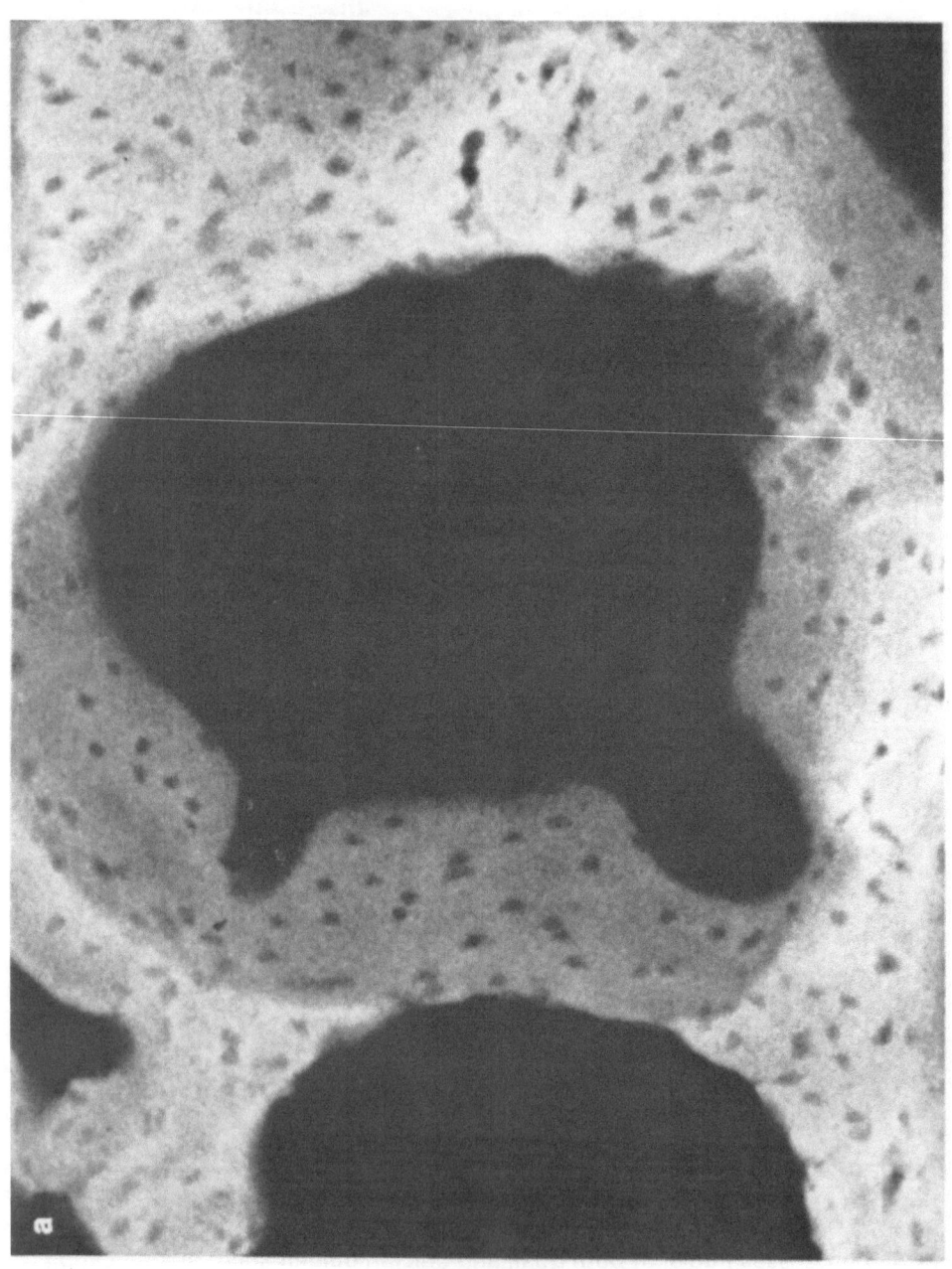

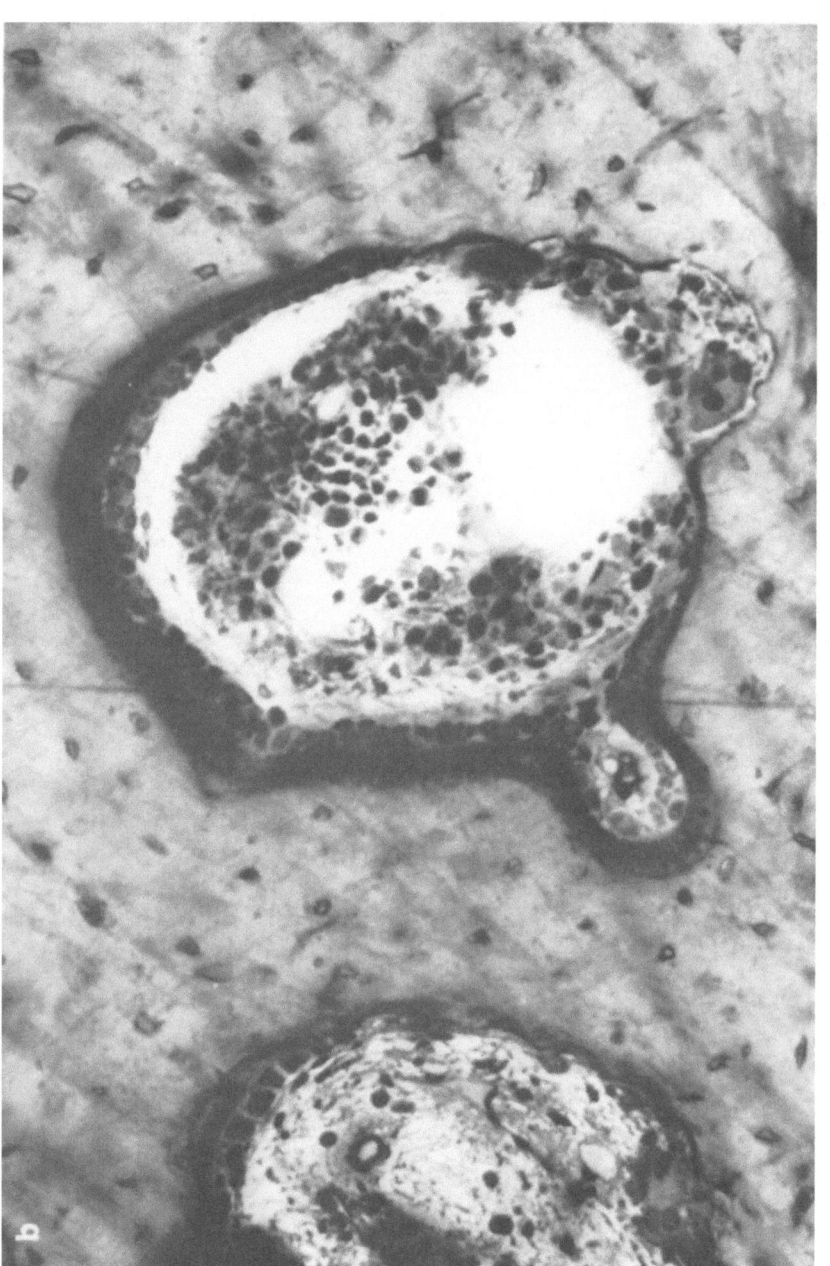

FIGURE 21. The microradiograph (a) and the stained, histological appearance (b) of a Haversian system in a mineralized bone section. Osteoclastic bone resorption is occurring in the lower right of the Haversian canal and bone formation in the upper left. The osteoclasts dedifferentiate and osteoblasts are differentiated from small progenitor cells (magnification ×500).

achieved by osteoclastic resorption of mineralized bone. An available source of calcium to maintain serum calcium levels would be impossible if osteoblastic bone formation were to be inevitably followed by resorption.

Similarly, if osteoblasts depended on the preexistence of osteoclasts, bone formation would be impossible in the majority of sites where, in fact, it does occur.

Chapter 3

Cortical and Trabecular Bone

Eighty percent of the skeleton consists of cortical bone, while twenty percent is trabecular; the percentages are of the wet or dry weight of the bone and do not include the soft-tissue or marrow spaces that make up part of the bone, particularly the trabecular or spongy bone. Evaluation of skeletal status, therefore, should be made on samples of bone in which the two types are present in approximately these two proportions. The majority of bone biopsy procedures include only trabecular bone and for this reason the quantitative results *must* be expected to be different from analyses which include both cortical and trabecular bone.

The differences between the two types of bone rest almost exclusively on the fact that trabecular bone has a larger surface-to-volume ratio than cortical bone (Table 1). As a result, although the activity per unit surface tends to be less in trabecular bone, the disappearance, in terms of percentage bone volume, is greater. From Table 1 it is apparent that there is three times as much surface per unit area or volume in trabecular compared with cortical bone. The variation is large; however, it

TABLE 1. Cortical and Trabecular Bone in the Anterior Iliac Crest

Group	Number of subjects	Cortical bone	Trabecular bone
Surface per unit area, mm/cm ^{2}			
Age-matched controls	94	55.0 ± 23.8^a	158.2 ± 63.1
Patients with osteoporosis	68	61.4 ± 14.8	149.6 ± 44.2
Percentage of bone in sample area			
Age-matched controls	92	68.5 ± 13.0	15.2 ± 6.8
Patients with osteoporosis	68	60.8 ± 12.4	11.6 ± 5.3

[a] Values are mean $\pm$ 1 SD.

TABLE 2. Rates of Loss of Bone in the Iliac Crest
from Ages 15 to 95

Females	
Cortical	0.552
Trabecular	0.189
Males	
Cortical	0.599
Trabecular	0.204

is probably true to say that there is no difference in the surface-to-volume ratio in normal and osteoporotic bone (Table 1).

If the percentage of bone is evaluated in a 50- to 70-year-old control population, that is, a group not presenting with osteoporosis, and compared with similar findings in a group with clinical evidence of the disease, it is evident that the loss of bone is only 12% greater in cortical bone compared with a 25% greater loss in trabecular bone (Table 1). Although the percentage rate of loss is greater in trabecular than cortical bone, the

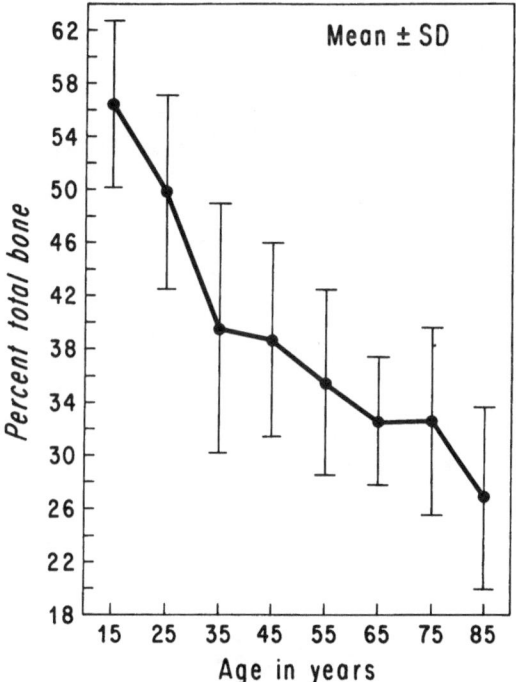

FIGURE 22. Videodensitometric assessment showing the loss of bone in the human rib with increasing age. Between ages 15 and 85 there has been a twofold decrease in bone mass within the periosteal boundary of the cortex including the marrow cavity and trabecular bone.

amount lost per unit time is slower than in cortical bone (Table 2). Figures 22 and 23a and b illustrate this point. In the rib, which is composed mainly of cortical bone, the volume of mineralized bone inside the periosteal boundary decreases from approximately 56 to 26% over an age span of 70 years, a twofold decrease or a loss of about half the bone (Figure 22). The same is true of the cortical part of the iliac crest; the values drop from approximately 80% at age 20 to 40% at age 90 (Figures 23a and b). Over the same age span, the trabecular bone

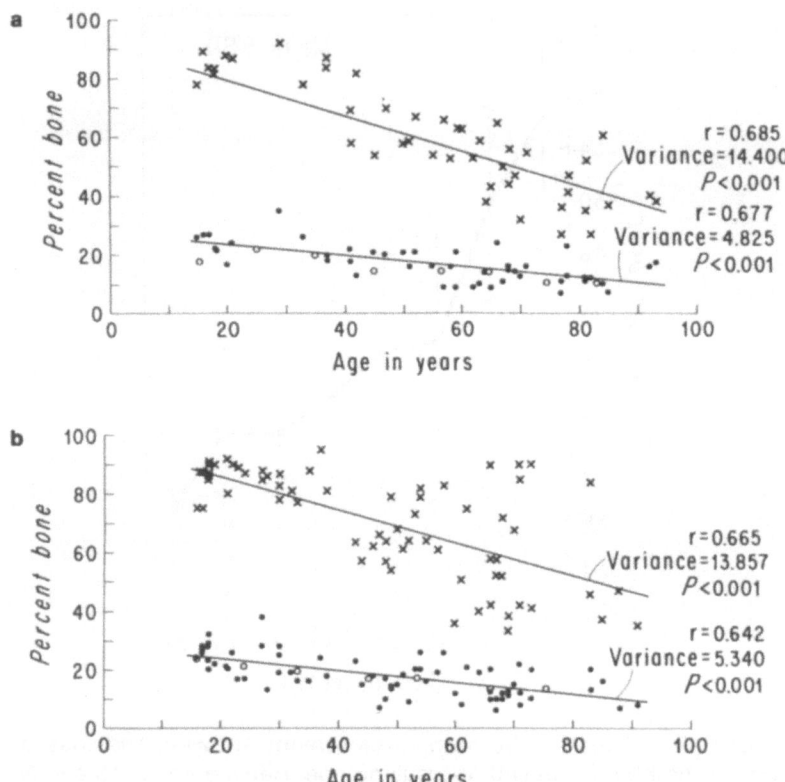

FIGURES 23a and b. Bone loss in the iliac crest in human beings with age. The slopes of the curves are given in Table 2. Percentage cortical and trabecular bone loss with age in females (a) and males (b). X = cortical bone, • = trabecular bone, o = trabecular bone by Meunier.

mass decreases from about 30 to 10%, a threefold decrease in volume which is greater than the percentage cortical bone loss, although it is apparent from Figures 23a and b and Table 2 that the rate of loss in trabecular bone is significantly less than the rate of loss of cortical bone. It is important to realize the significance of these differences; the percentage loss of bone will be reflected in the radiographic changes and in the strength of the bone, and since two-thirds of trabecular bone disappears with increasing age, it is in predominantly trabecular bones, such as the vertebrae and the femoral head and neck, that radiographic changes can be most easily and quickly seen. On the other hand, since the absolute rate of loss is less, the cellular activity per unit surface can be expected to be less, and indeed it is; if, for example, bone formation, in terms of the bone surface activity, is measured in trabecular and cortical areas separately, the cortical bone values lie between 3.5 and 6%, while in the trabecular area of the same series of biopsy samples, the values are between 1.5 and 2.5% (Figure 24). There is also a sugges-

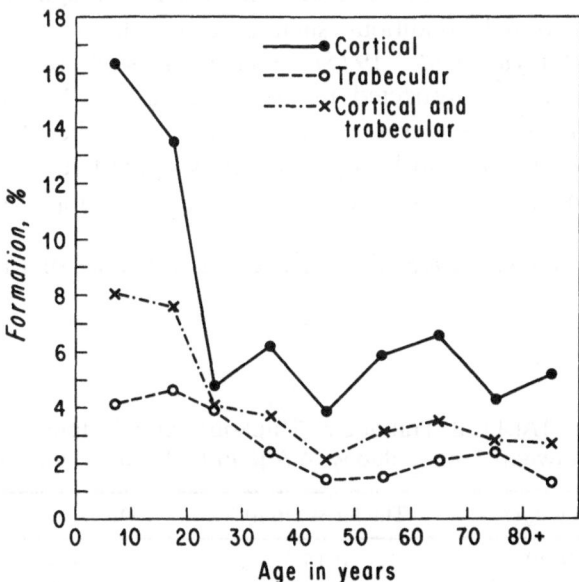

FIGURE 24. Bone formation measured by quantitative microradiography in iliac crest biopsies in cortical and trabecular bone. The values are the percentage of the total surface occupied by formation of bone. ●————● = cortical, o————o = trabecular, ×—·—× = cortical and trabecular.

tion that there may be quantitative differences in the two types of bone. The volume of trabecular bone decreases relatively rapidly initially and later shows almost no change with increase in age, while cortical bone does not start to show a significant loss until approximately age 40; therefore, at early ages trabecular bone will more nearly represent total skeletal changes than at later ages, when this type of bone is relatively inactive, while cortical bone will demonstrate a greater cellular activity in later years. There is no reduction in thickness in trabeculae accompanying the decrease in mass of trabecular bone (Table 3) (Wakamatsu and Sissons, 1969). The decrease occurs by complete loss of trabeculae so that they become less frequent, with wider spaces between them. Measurements of trabecular thickness, therefore, do not reflect bone loss, although they may reflect abnormal conditions such as osteosclerosis (Connor *et al.*, 1974; Kyle *et al.*, 1975). It is the loss of trabeculae, in sequence, that is reflected in the Singh index (Singh *et al.*, 1972). As age increases there is a loss of trabeculae in the femoral head that can be approximately quantitated to give an indication of bone loss and that is related to symptoms of osteoporosis.

As a consequence, the surface per unit area of trabecular

TABLE 3. Trabecular Thickness and Distance
between Trabeculae with Age in Males and Females[a]

Age (yr)	Thickness (mm)	Distance (mm)
20–29	0.15	0.94
30–39	0.15	0.99
40–49	0.14	0.97
50–59	0.13	1.05
60–69	0.13	1.14
70–100	0.14	1.16

[a] From Wakamatsu and Sissons, 1969.

bone does not increase significantly with age, as seen in Table 1, and although there will be a few individual trabeculae that are thinner (as they are in the process of being resorbed), the average width remains the same.

Cortical bone loss occurs by an absolute loss of bone from the endosteal surface, and to a lesser extent by an increase in the number of holes in the cortex. For this reason measurements of the amount of bone in an area, defined as cortex by being made up of compact bone, will show only a small decrease with age and a small difference between normal and osteoporotic individuals (Table 1). If, on the other hand, a normal cortex is defined by a line that separates bone containing a greater percentage of bone than soft tissue from bone that is more than half made up of soft tissue, and if the width of the cortex is defined as the width of bone between this line and the periosteum, then normal average cortical thickness in 15- to 25-year-old healthy individuals can be measured. If it is assumed only that an older person had a cortical thickness at age 20 that was similar to this figure, the loss of bone from the endosteal surface can be evaluated by including in the "cortex" the endosteal bone area that has been lost and now consists of trabecular bone. In this way the true loss of cortical bone, including the endosteal disappearance of bone and the increased porosity, can be measured, as in Figures 23a and b.

Because the majority of bone loss occurs from cortical bone, it is therefore necessary to include cortical bone in any analysis of bone cell activity both because it represents a majority of the skeleton and because this is where bone is being lost and where cell activity is highest in individuals over age 50, which is the age at which most symptoms occur as a result of metabolic bone disease. It is also evident that the differences between the two types of bone are responsible for the different results reported in various analyses of bone biopsies. Merz, Meunier, and Bordier all report a decrease in bone formation with increasing age (Bordier et al., 1964; Merz and Schenk, 1970; Meunier et al., 1973a), a finding which is also true of trabecular bone analyzed by the combined quantitative microradiographic and histological techniques as shown in Figure 23a and b. It is unfortunate that, in some instances, these authors and other investigators regard the difference as being the result of the method of analysis, inferring that one or the other technique must be in error. The previous discussion and the accompanying data show that it is the type of bone that is analyzed that explains the difference in the data and further cautions against the interpretation of skeletal metabolism in the light of data from trabecular bone only.

Chapter 4

The Bone Biopsy

Most biopsy procedures suffer from two disadvantages; the first is that they are invasive, with the possible consequences of pain, bleeding, and infection, while the second concerns the question of how representative the specimen is of the whole tissue. Both difficulties can be partially overcome; the first by the use of a careful surgical procedure in which the muscle is cut as little as possible, while the infection and bleeding are controlled by antibiotics and packing or hemostasis if necessary. The question of variation from site to site in the body can be answered in two ways; the first is to assume that in metabolic and systemic diseases all parts of the tissue will be affected, if not equally at least proportionally, while the other approach is to sample a reasonable number of different parts of the tissue to ascertain the correctness of the assumption. Since the majority of tissues are made up of component parts that differ in both structure and function (i.e., the kidney is made up of cortex and medulla, while bone can be separated into trabecular or spongy bone and cortical or compact bone) it is necessary to sample all component parts in the proportion in which they occur in the body to obtain a representative sample of the organ. Although it is obvious, of course, that if only part of the tissue is of interest, then only that part needs to be sampled.

Despite the disadvantages, the information derived from tissue biopsies can be obtained in no other way than to observe the tissue itself. For example, a decrease in density on X ray may be the result of excessive removal of bone or inadequate bone deposition. While measurements of the amount of calcium in the urine and of vitamin D metabolites to evaluate calcium absorption and other methods may be applied to gain further insight into the abnormal bone status, a bone biopsy is frequently necessary in order to understand precisely the nature of the skeletal abnormality.

It is probably worthwhile to illustrate this point now with a case report: a 58-year-old female with a history of mild hypercalcemia documented 12 years previous to being seen at hospital X and at intervals thereafter. It was, however, not known whether hypercalcemia existed previously. The patient developed a fracture of a lumbar vertebra and was admitted for study. The hypercalcemia had always been accompanied by hypophosphatemia, and although primary hyperparathyroidism was suspected, no neck exploration was carried out because of the mildness of the hypercalcemia and the disinclination of the patient to undergo surgery. At the time of the fracture when osteoporosis was diagnosed, the hypophosphatemia had persisted and was exaggerated and the urinary calcium was markedly decreased (98 mg/24 h). At this time also the hypercalcemia had reverted to hypocalcemia (8.1 mg/dl). An assay for immunoreactive parathyroid hormone was carried out and the value was found to be 150 μleq/ml, a value that fell well above normal. The question then arose as to why the patient did not present with the characteristic bone radiographic signs of hyperparathyroidism such as subperiosteal erosion of the phalanges and why the serum calcium was low rather than high. A bone biopsy revealed that bone mass was markedly decreased, as would be expected in a patient with osteoporosis and hyperparathyroidism, while the more important and unique finding of increased amount of bone surface covered by unmineralized osteoid tissue explained the more unusual aspects of the case. The serum phosphate had been low enough, coupled with the only mild elevation of serum calcium, to cause a failure of mineralization of bone. Osteoclastic resorption had continued as long as mineralized tissue was available but as osteoid surfaces increased to the values of 82% seen in the biopsy, the removal of mineralized bone decreased, since osteoclasts are in most instances inhibited from resorbing matrix containing no mineral. This resulted in a decreased urinary calcium, a fall in serum calcium which further stimulated the parathyroid gland activity, resulting in exaggerated renal effect and a further fall in serum phosphate. Despite the attempt of the parathyroids to maintain calcium homeostasis, this proved impossible because of the significant accumulation of osteoid which effectively sealed off the bone from the influence of the parathyroids. The case would have been most puzzling to interpret without the information gained from the bone biopsy.

PROCEDURE FOR TAKING A BONE BIOPSY

The first point to be established is whether or not a bone biopsy is necessary. A patient with all the clinical and biochemical signs of osteomalacia such as bone pain, pseudofractures, a high alkaline phosphatase, and a low serum phosphate will not profit to any great extent from a bone biopsy, which will merely confirm the presence of excess amounts of osteoid. A jejunal biopsy or measurement of vitamin D metabolites to investigate the cause of the osteomalacia will be more worthwhile. Bone biopsy is indicated most frequently in instances where borderline biochemical values are reported and the clinical findings are not clear-cut. Since the primary function of the skeleton is to provide calcium under the direction of the parathyroid glands, the overwhelming majority of patients with osteomalacia will have underlying osteoporosis, and in areas of the world where there is vitamin D deficiency, osteomalacia may accompany what clinically appears as osteoporosis. A biopsy is helpful in such instances since the osteomalacia, if it exists, must first be corrected before the osteoporosis can be treated and before calcium homeostasis can be expected to be maintained.

If a suspicious lesion is seen on X ray and cannot be diagnosed, a biopsy is generally carried out to identify the lesion. If the appearance on X ray suggests a serious problem, a biopsy is mandatory, and a small piece of bone or cartilage will generally suffice. A Craig needle is generally used and a closed biopsy is performed if possible. The biopsy can be taken under local anesthesia using 2% Xylocaine and with anterior, posterior, and lateral X rays to allow for exact positioning of the needle at the site of the lesion (Evarts, 1975). In some areas a closed biopsy is not suggested but rather an open biopsy is called for because of the risk of damaging adjacent structures: In the region of T_1 to T_9 the parietal pleura is adjacent to the vertebrae and the azygous and the hemiazygous venous systems are close to the vertebral bodies above T_{10} (Evarts, 1975; Debnam and Staple, 1975a). Pneumothorax has resulted from closed trephine biopsies of the dorsal spine (Debnam and Staple, 1975a).

Biopsy of long bones, particularly the primary weight-bearing bones, should be undertaken with great reserve because even the small defect produced by the Craig needle will weaken the bone seemingly out of all proportion to the size of the hole.

Diagnosis of the biopsy can be made using frozen or demineralized paraffin-embedded procedures. Alternatively, soft-tissue smears can be made of tumor tissue to identify the lesion seen on X ray (Thommesen and Frederiksen, 1976). In general the technique is useful in identification of the lesion. However, up to 30% of unsuccessful biopsies have been reported, "unsuccessful" being described as the failure of the diagnosis made from the biopsy to be supported by any other evidence (Debnam and Staple, 1975b). Flat-bone biopsies tend to be less successful diagnostically, since only small samples of tissue can be obtained; in one reported series only three out of nine bone biopsies proved useful, however, it is not possible to decide if the site of the biopsy or the degree of involvement of those bones (scapula, humerus, clavicle) was at fault (Debnam and Staple, 1975b).

Apart from the usefulness of a bone biopsy for diagnostic purposes, biopsies have been used extensively to evaluate the bone tissue abnormalities characteristic of certain diseases. In such instances the clinical presentation is generally clear; a comparison of bone taken from patients with known bone disease with bone from a control population provides information regarding the deviation from normal that results in the clinical symptoms.

A third use that has become more frequent in recent years is to evaluate the effects of various therapeutic regimes on bone, the advantage being that changes in bone formation and resorption will result in decreases or increases in bone mass that can be evaluated at short intervals long before radiographic changes are seen. In most bone disease bone loss is the cause of the pain and disability and it is generally the aim of the therapy to increase bone mass back toward normal and to a state where fracture will not occur. Bone biopsies can also be used to evaluate the effect of therapy and predict the long-term effects of such therapy before they become evident by X ray or a decreased fracture rate.

THE SITE OF THE BIOPSY

Two sites for biopsy have been used almost exclusively, the rib and the iliac crest. The rib is less satisfactory as a biopsy site because it results in what is essentially a fracture, with consequent pain that persists for some time. In addition, the rib contains a somewhat larger proportion of cortical to trabecular bone than is representative of the skeleton as a whole.

Rib biopsies have been used by Frost and co-workers, the majority of the material being obtained as a result of a thoracotomy or by biopsy (Frost and Villanueva, 1961; Barer and Jowsey, 1967). Trephine biopsies and sections of ribs have been used in animal studies in order to be able to take a number of similar samples, i.e., more than two, from an anatomically identical bone (Cabanela and Jowsey, 1974; Little, 1972). Full sections of the rib are preferable to smaller biopsies since the pain comes from the two fractured ends of the bone rubbing together. Sections should also be taken from the same side so that the animal or person can comfortably lie on the other intact side. Alternatively, in animals, sections can be taken from the dorsal ribs adjacent to the spinal column (Cabanela and Jowsey, 1974). In this way many specimens can be taken at frequent intervals without any complications, such as fracture repair involving subsequent biopsies. Six biopsies have been taken in adult dogs in this manner with no complications, and more were possible, provided alternate ribs are left intact attached to the spine in order to prevent collapse of the rib cage and consequent respiratory problems. Nevertheless, it is obvious to orthopedic surgeons who have had experience with rib biopsies and with iliac crest biopsies that the former hold more risk, due to a possible pneumothorax, and they can also be significantly more painful than the latter. The rib also has the disadvantage that it is composed largely of cortical bone, containing little trabecular bone (Figure 25).

The iliac crest is almost universally used because here a biopsy does not result in a fracture, the proportion of trabecular to cortical bone is similar to that in the whole skeleton, and the procedure can be almost painless. The site of biopsy, the size of the trephine used, and the area of bone analyzed varies a great deal (Table 4). The majority of investigators use a trephine which varies in size between 3.0 mm in diameter, such as that used by Smirnov and Byers, and 7.5 mm in diameter, as used by Jowsey (Smirnov and Baranov, 1971; Byers and Smith, 1967; Johnson et al., 1977). Biopsies of the iliac crest are generally transilial and taken below the iliac crest, however, some investigators take biopsies vertically through the iliac crest (Figure 26). There is also variation in the type of bone used as well as in the method of preparing the sections. Probably the size of

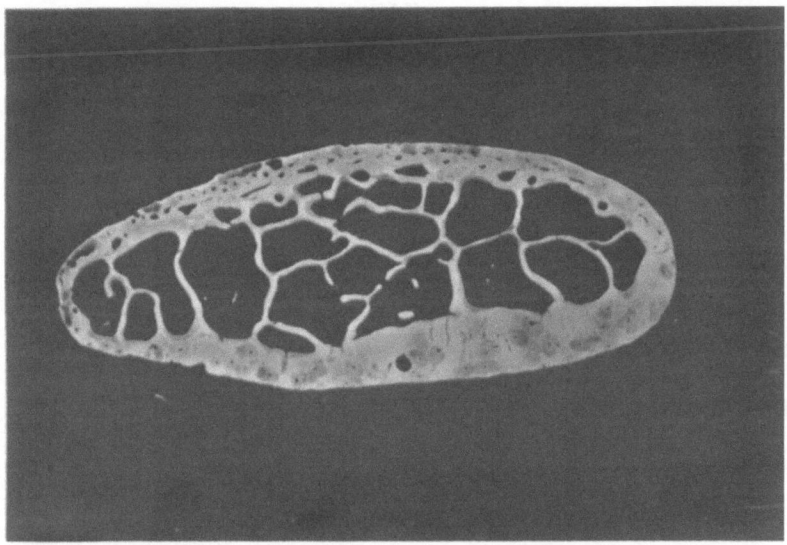

FIGURE 25. Microradiograph of a cross section of a rib of a normal adult human being. The majority of the bone is cortical and consists of secondary Haversian systems (magnification ×7).

the biopsy and the type of bone, trabecular as compared with trabecular and cortical, are the most important variations and account for the majority of differences between values obtained by different investigators. It is worthwhile describing the different techniques used by investigators since different bone samples will yield results that must be expected to differ.

The trephine used by Smirov and Baranov (1971) is 3 mm in diameter and has a sharp cutting edge. It is perhaps unique in that the cutting cylinder is made of two half-cylinders which fit together by means of a groove in the distal portion, the whole fitting into a thin-walled tube which is slightly shorter than the cutting cylinder. In this way the thin-walled tube can be slipped off the cylinders and the cylinders are parted to free the biopsy. Since the specimen is so slender and potentially long, depending on the thickness of the iliac crest (which may be over 1.0 or 2.0

TABLE 4

Authors	Trephine diameter (mm)	Area of bone	Type of bone	Analysis
Smirnov and Baranov (1971)	3.0	Anterior and/or transilial		—
Fornasier and Vilaghy (1973)	3.0	Posterior and/or transilial		Unmineralized or demineralized
Sacker and Nordin (1954)	5.0	Vertical		—
Duursma et al. (1969)	5.0	Vertical		Mineralized and demineralized
Woods et al. (1968)	5.0	Vertical	Trabecular	Mineralized
Sherrard et al. (1974)	4.0	Vertical	Trabecular	
Bordier et al. (1964)	6.0	Transilial	Trabecular	Mineralized
Courpron et al. (1974)	6.0	Transilial	Trabecular	Mineralized
Byers and Smith (1967)	7.2	Transilial	Trabecular	Microradiographs and mineralized
Teitelbaum et al. (1976b)	5.0	Transilial	Cortical and trabecular	Mineralized
Johnson et al. (1977) Jowsey et al. (1971)	7.5–10.0	Transilial	Cortical and trabecular	Mineralized and microradiographs

cm from cortex to cortex) the separation of the cylinder is no doubt necessary to prevent the specimen of tissue from collapsing as it would if pushed out with a solid rod. The samples are similar to those depicted in Figure 26c but are only 3 mm in diameter. The procedure has been free of complications. Although over one hundred biopsies have been taken, no further data have

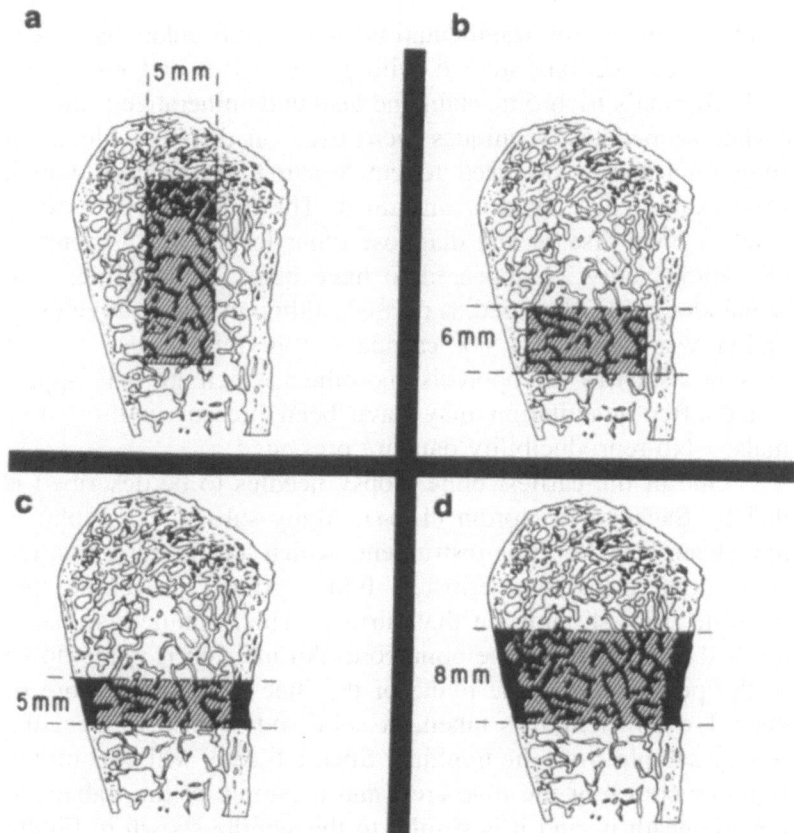

FIGURE 26. Diagram to show the various methods of taking a bone biopsy of the iliac crest and the different areas analyzed by different investigators. (a) Superior iliac crest biopsy. (b–d) Transilial biopsies.

come to light regarding the use of the biopsies, repeatability, etc. Possibily those reports exist in the Russian literature since Smirnov is from the USSR.

Fornasier (Fornasier and Vilaghy, 1973) uses a 3 mm diameter needle also, but without the asset of the split cylinder described by Smirnov. Nevertheless, only 12% of the biopsies showed collapse or fragmentation of the trabeculae. Both demineralized sections stained with hematoxylin and eosin and with Masson's trichrome stain and also undemineralized, methacrylate embedded techniques were used on different blocks; a Jung microtome was used to cut 8 μm thick sections which were examined, stained or unstained. The material was used to confirm bone disease and diagnose other lesions. In a group of 68 patients only 23 appeared to have bone abnormalities, the remainder being classified as normal, although quantitative evaluation was apparently not carried out in this series, so that disorders such as osteoporosis and others which are only appreciated after quantitation may have been present in the "normals." No reproducibility data are presented.

One of the earliest bone biopsy needles to be described is that by Sacker and Nordin (1954). Many subsequent trephines have been based on this instrument, which has an outer toothed sleeve that grips the periosteal bone surface, preventing the trephine from slipping on that surface. The trephine also has a toothed end and takes the bone core. An incision is made down to the periosteum in the plane of the iliac spine and a core of bone 1 cm in length is taken. A solid rod is used to eject the biopsy sample from the trephine. Such a biopsy will contain the superior cortex of the iliac crest and a sample of the trabecular bone beneath it, and it is similar to the sample shown in Figure 26a.

Duursma and colleagues have used a somewhat different type of biopsy trephine based on one used by Dekker (Duursma et al., 1969; Dekker et al., 1968). A base cylinder of 7 mm in diameter ends in a circle, five-sixths of which contains a serrated blade that can be maneuvered at 90° to the cylinder or extended outside the cylinder by means of a lever. The trephine itself is 7.0 mm in external diameter and 5.0 mm in internal diameter and is used to take a vertical biopsy through a small incision 2 cm dorsal to the superior iliac spine. The base saw is then used to cut the base of a 2 cm long plug which is then ejected. After fixation the specimen is cut in half lengthwise, and both demineralized and undemineralized methacrylate sections are cut and stained. The sample is of the type shown in Figure 26a but contains the outer cortex. No reproducibility data are given.

A 5 mm diameter trephine is also used by Woods and colleagues (Woods *et al.*, 1968). An incision is made down to the periosteum of the ilium in the plane of the iliac crest and a biopsy is taken under local anesthesia by a technique developed by Williams and Nicholson (1963). The trabecular bone is separated from the outer cortex and embedded by the double-embedding technique and 5 μm thick sections are cut and stained. The bone biopsy is of the area illustrated in Figure 26a. The major early use of the method was to measure osteoid width thickness and the extent of the bone surface covered by osteoid; both are reflections of osteomalacia. The authors used polarized light and measured birefringent lamellae of collagen and a Chalkey point array graticule that has 25 points for each field measured. By using polarized light any variation resulting from oblique sections or surfaces is eliminated, since obliquity will be reflected in the width rather than in the number of alternate bands of polarized lamellae of osteoid. A comparison of a 10- and 40-fold magnification indicated that at 10-fold magnification only osteoid of 1 μm in thickness was not seen, and this was considered insignificant. Evaluation of the thickness of the osteoid and the length of surface covered by osteoid were repeated by a single observer and also by two observers, and the variance was small. The number of fields that was needed to obtain consistent values was measured in four sections, and it was found that there was no increase in accuracy achieved by measuring more than 10 fields. In converting the number of bright lines to micrometers of osteoid, a perpendicular surface that can be identified at high power by microscopy showed that a bright and dark band were each 2 μm in thickness. In normal bone up to three bright bands were seen, equivalent to 12 μm of osteoid, although osteoid up to 50 μm wide can be seen in oblique surfaces of bone. The technique is no doubt accurate and the authors have not troubled to evaluate observer error and repeatability. The differences between the thickness of osteoid and particularly the extent of surface covered by osteoid is large when normal and clinically osteomalacic patients are compared. The only shortcoming of the method is the limitation of sensitivity resulting from the manner of measuring alternating bands of birefringence. The resolution is 4 μm, that is, in normal bone 0–3 bands only can be seen, which cover dimensions of 0–20 μm if direct measurements are made using a calibrated eyepiece. Thus the difference between the variations seen in normal individuals may be invisible. Cell populations have also been evaluated by these authors using a similar technique.

Sherrard (Sherrard *et al.*, 1974) also takes a vertical bone biopsy, but in contrast to Nordin and Sacket and to Woods, he eliminates the external cortex in his evaluation of bone morphometry, and the diameter of the core is only 0.4 cm (Figure 26a). Mineralized sections are made and stained by the Goldner stain, and the amount of osteoid and forming and resorbing surfaces are evaluated quantitatively. The major group studied by these investigators has been patients with chronic uremia and renal osteodystrophy. The patients vary from mildly affected to more severely affected individuals, the latter showing morphological signs of osteitis fibrosa. The data on bone formation are difficult to understand since the surface occupied by bone formation is from two to four times normal, and bone formation rate calculated from surface and tetracycline data is twice normal, although bone resorption values are normal and bone volume is decreased or normal (Table 5). The investigators suggest that bone resorption rate must be increased to account for this discrepancy. However, it is also likely that the estimation of bone formation surfaces are at fault; a value of 79% for percentage bone formation surface in osteomalacia is above any value reported in osteomalacia or renal osteodystrophy by other investigators. These investigators use the presence of osteoid to evaluate bone formation (Sherrard *et al.*, 1974), and in any

TABLE 5. Bone Morphometry in Patients with Chronic Uremia[a]

	Normal	Mild bone abnormality	Malacic bone
Volume bone (% tissue area)	22.8 ± 8.1	16.6 ± 4.6[b]	30.8 ± 19.8
Forming surface (% total surface)	16.9 ± 7.2	34.8 ± 9.9[b]	79.3 ± 9.8[b]
Resorbing surface (% total surface)	4.9 ± 3.3	5.7 ± 1.8	4.9 ± 2.0
Bone formation rate ($mm^3/mm^3/day \times 10^{-4}$)	1.88 ± 1.9	2.87 ± 1.13	3.25 ± 2.29

[a] From Sherrard et al., 1973. All values are mean ± SD.
[b] Significant difference from normal at $P < 0.001$.

disease characterized by lack of of mineralization this value will be high and not representative of active osteoblastic bone formation. Indeed, osteomalacia has generally been associated with a decreased bone formation level, particularly when seen as the result of chronic disease (Kelly et al., 1965).

A 6.0 mm transilial anterior iliac crest biopsy taken 2 cm behind the superior spine is used by Bordier who developed the trephine that includes as a primary procedure, after a small skin incision, the separation of the muscles over the lateral surface of the iliac crest by means of a short angled but pointed obturator. The specimen is partially demineralized for 4–8 h in 10% nitric acid. This procedure renders the section easy to cut without removing all the bone mineral. Sections 5 μm thick are cut and stained by the Goldner stain or with toluidine, and the trabecular bone is analyzed in two nonconsecutive sections, cortical bone being deliberately excluded (Figure 26b) (Bordier et al., 1964). Approximately eight areas, defined by a Zeiss grid, are evaluated in each section, and the bone volume is measured by counting the number of times the lines (six per grid) intersect with a bone surface. In each biopsy about 1200 intersections are measured. A modified Zeiss grid (no. II) with finite ends to the

six parallel lines is used for evaluation of resorption or formation.

Resorption is evaluated by measuring the resorption surface
covered with osteoclasts, while formation is a measure of osteoid covered by active osteoblasts. Bordier therefore avoids
any error made by confusing "active" osteoid, which is in the
process of bone matrix deposition, and "inactive" osteoid,
where formation of osteoid has ceased but it has remained unmineralized. Bordier also measured the calcification front; this
is a subjective evaluation of the presence or absence of the
granular border between osteoid and mineralized bone and is
normally present in 80% of the osteoid border surface (Bordier
and Tun Chot, 1973). Solochrome cyanine has proved unreli-
able (Bordier and Tun Chot, 1973), probably because the procedure involves immersing the sections in solutions of low pH that
remove recently deposited mineral and therefore would be expected to remove variably the mineralization front. The same
may be true of the toluidine blue staining procedure carried out
at pH 2.8.

Bordier also measures "inactive" resorption, a term which
might better be termed "previous" resorption, since it refers to
a resorption surface which is no longer resorbing and where
bone formation has not yet taken place. Since it is not possible
to tell when the resorption stopped, measurement of "inactive"
resorption does not reflect the metabolic status of the bone at the
time of biopsy, however, it may be a useful parameter in reflecting a past history of a bone abnormality.

Repeatability of the method of Bordier is poor, probably
because only trabecular bone is evaluated but largely because of
the small size of the biopsy (Figure 27) (Table 6); methods of
analysis of small biopsies and of trabecular bone are also poor
(Table 7). A similar biopsy is used by Meunier et al., (1973b)
and has a relatively poor repeatability for bone resorption and
formation, although this investigator and his colleagues have
concentrated their investigations largely on the evaluation of
bone porosity, which shows good repeatability (Courpron et al.,

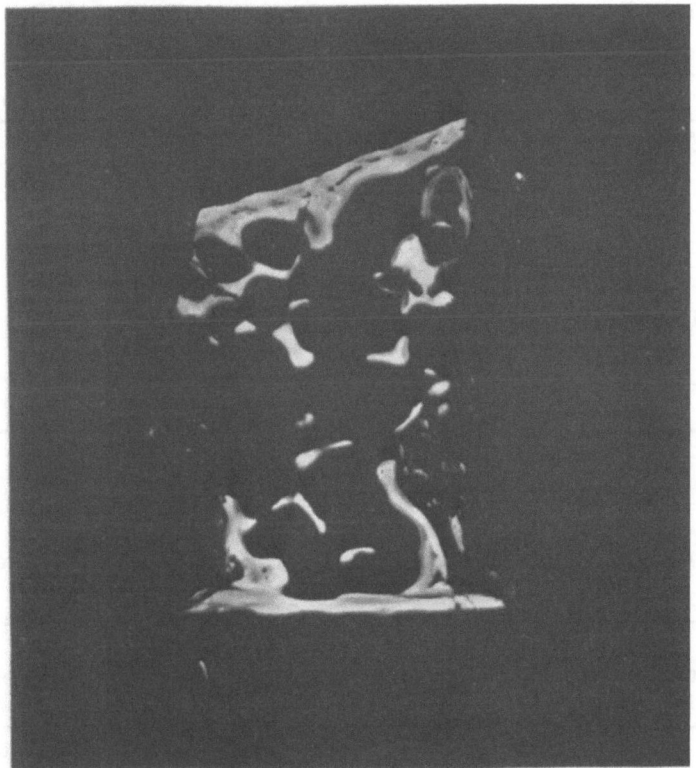

FIGURE 27. Microradiograph of a small 5 mm diameter biopsy. The volume of bone in an 8 mm diameter specimen is 2.5 times as great as one that is 5 mm in diameter (magnification × 7).

1974). Evaluations of porosity are termed trabecular bone volume, since only trabecular bone is analyzed (Figure 28).

An analysis of repeatability and a general idea of the reliability of the method is also given by Byers and Smith who use a 7.2 mm diameter trephine and transilial biopsy (Byers and Smith, 1967). The specimen includes both the internal and the external cortex and is similar to the area shown in Figure 26d but smaller. Undecalcified and demineralized specimens are

TABLE 6. Repeatability of Measurements in Trabecular Bone
Analyzed in a 5-mm-Diameter Biopsy[a]

	First time	Second time
Osteoid volume		
(% bone tissue)	0.6	3.2
Osteoid surface		
(% total surface)	15.3	19.6
Calcification front		
(% osteoid surface)	54.0	66.0
Total resorption surface		
(% cancellous bone surface)	8.7	10.5
Osteocytic osteolysis		
(% total lacunae)	7.44	1.8

[a] From Bordier et al., 1972.

TABLE 7. Repeatability of Bone Morphometry Values by Three
Investigators Using Biopsies of Different Sizes

Study No.[a]	Size of trephine (mm)	Average Δ[b]	Standard deviation of Δ	Standard error of Δ	Number of trials
1	5	3.3	3.7	1.6	6
2	5	1.2	1.3	0.4	10
3	9	1.9	1.7	0.6	8
2	9	0.6	0.4	0.1	22

[a] Unpublished data.
[b] Δ = Difference

used depending on the investigation. Formation is identified by
the presence of osteoid tissue and resorption by microradiographic analyses.

The first question asked by these authors was whether a
bone biopsy could identify the bone disease process or processes
in primary hyperparathyroidism with more accuracy than was
indicated by radiographic methods. In a group of 24 patients

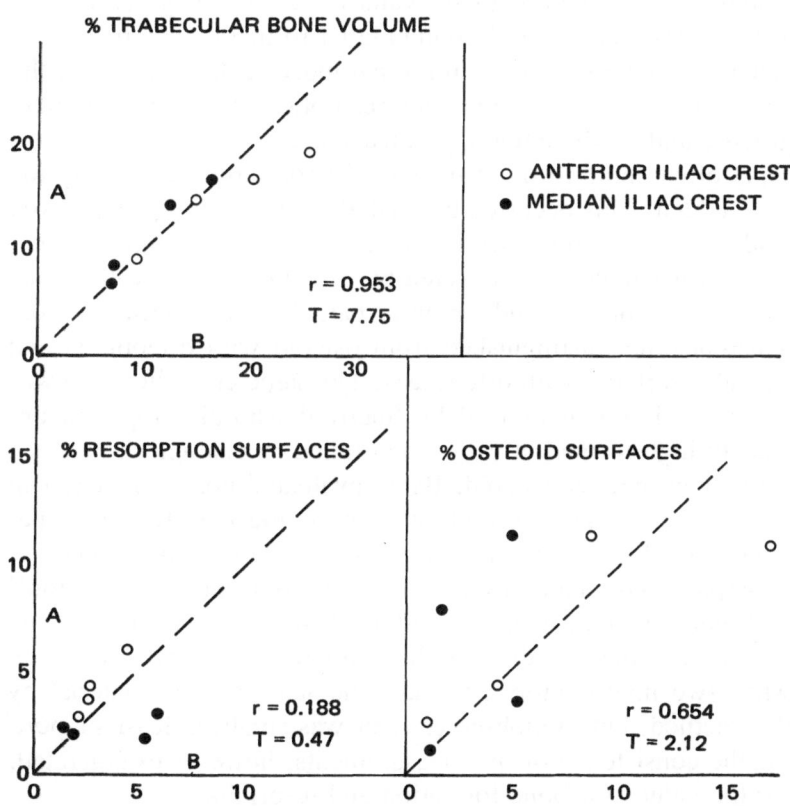

FIGURE 28. Repeatability in eight transilial biopsies in which only trabecular bone was analyzed. The bone volume shows good repeatability, but resorption and osteoid surfaces are not as good. The dotted line is the line of equality. From Meunier and Edouard (1973). o = anterior iliac crest, ● = median iliac crest.

with hyperparathyroidism, 13 had no X-ray evidence of bone disease while having other evidence of disturbed parathyroid function such as renal stones or hypercalcemia. Using a grid and a point count system that gave values as a percentage of total intercepts, Byers and Smith found higher formation and resorption values in the patients than in normal individuals. In general, the values for both formation and resorption were high in both groups, and as the authors pointed out the percentage of intercepts often came to more than 100 if formation and resorption were added. This occurred because the microradiograph showed evidence of resorption while the same area, under light microscopy, was shown to be covered by osteoid. Osteoid with no associated osteoblasts and irregular calcified bone surfaces were apparently not distinguished from osteoid with osteoblasts and irregular surfaces with osteoclasts. The same error therefore was encouraged as experienced by Sherrard who also reported unusually high formation values and failed to distinguish between active and inactive osteoid. Byers evaluated normal material in the same way and "resorption" was found elevated in all patients including the 13 who showed no radiological evidence of hyperparathyroidism. In addition, osteoid and "resorption" both correlated with the logarithm of alkaline phosphatase and total 24-h urinary hydroxyproline. Interobserver error was high when two investigators evaluated the same normal material by this method, but intraobserver error was small, at least supporting the consistency of the measurements, however exaggerated, for the values for bone formation and resorption.

Cortical bone, in addition to trabecular bone, is evaluated by three investigators, Frost, Teitelbaum, and Jowsey (Frost, 1958; Teitelbaum et al., 1976b; Jowsey et al., 1965). Rib biopsies have not, on the whole, met with much success because of the discomfort and potential danger of a pneumothorax, as already mentioned. The majority of samples of rib reported in the literature have come from autopsy cases or from patients requiring a thoracotomy in the process of a surgical procedure (Landeros and Frost, 1964; Barer and Jowsey, 1967). Bone resorption and formation appear to occur at a relatively unchanged level with age in bone from this area. In addition, rib bone biopsy in patients not requiring surgery is difficult to justify, and for this reason the iliac crest has been the biopsy site chosen by most investigators.

A transilial biopsy of the iliac crest 0.5 mm in diameter is the method preferred by Teitelbaum, and the analysis includes both external and internal cortices (Teitelbaum et al., 1976b). The sample area is represented by the diagram in Figure 26c. Methacrylate-undemineralized specimens are cut with a microtome and stained by the Goldner technique. Bone mass is evaluated using cortical thickness and porosity, bone formation by the presence of osteoblasts, and bone resorption by the presence of osteoclasts. Active and inactive osteoid is also evaluated. The results are expressed as the number of cells per square millimeter of the section (osteoclasts and osteoblasts) or as a percentage of surface occupied by osteoid or of cortex occupied by space. The data have been reported separately for cortical and trabecular bone, and it has therefore been possible to evaluate the relative levels of resorption and formation occurring in these

TABLE 8. Serum Parathyroid Hormone (iPTH) and Osteoclastic
Bone Resorption in Cortical and Trabecular Bone
from Patients with Osteoporosis[a]

	Trabecular osteoclasts per square millimeter	Cortical osteoclasts per square millimeter
iPTH > 10 μleq/ml	0.65 ± 0.48	6.7 ± 1.5
iPTH < 10 μleq/ml	0.41 ± 0.45	0.46 ± 0.29
	NS[b]	$p < .005$

[a] From Teitelbaum et al., 1976a. Values are mean ± SD.
[b] Not significant: trabecular osteoclasts with iPTH > 10 to trabecular osteoclasts with iPTH < 10.

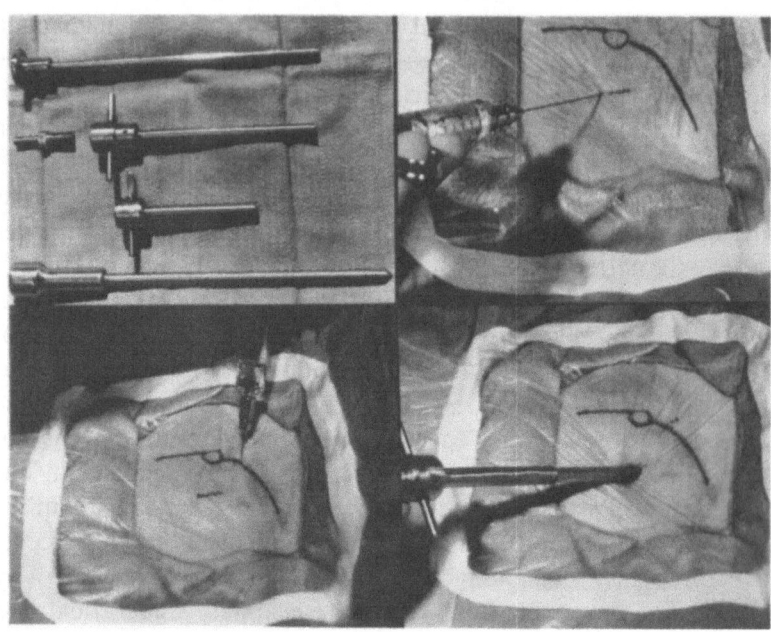

FIGURE 29. Bone biopsy needle and surgical procedure for taking an iliac crest biopsy, as used at the Mayo Clinic. In the upper left is shown the blunt extractor, the trephine with threaded extension for attachment to a power tool, the outer sleeve, and the pointed obturator for separating the tissue over the outer cortex of the ilium. In the upper right the outer aspect of the ilium is locally anesthetized, the line indicates the margin of the iliac crest. In the lower left the inner aspect of the ilium is anesthetized locally and in the lower right, the pointed obturator is inserted through a 1 cm skin incision. From Johnson *et al.*, 1977.

two areas of the biopsy. It is particularly relevant to a discussion of both cortical and trabecular bone and to analyses of the importance of the proportion of these two types of bone in a biopsy that cortical bone resorption was elevated in the patients with increased parathyroid hormone activity and not in those with parathyroid levels within the normal range (Table 8). Bone resorption in trabecular bone was not significantly increased.

Jowsey has used an 8.0 or a 7.5 mm diameter trephine to obtain a transilial biopsy of the iliac crest. The size of the biopsy was optimum, a larger one, 1.5 mm in diameter, providing no additional data and a 5 mm diameter biopsy demonstrating poor repeatability (Table 7). The biopsy can be obtained by a percutaneous method under local anesthesia (Johnson *et al.*, 1977) (Figure 29). The biopsy contains both external and internal cortices (Figure 30). The specimen is embedded in methacrylate and a microradiograph is made of a section 100

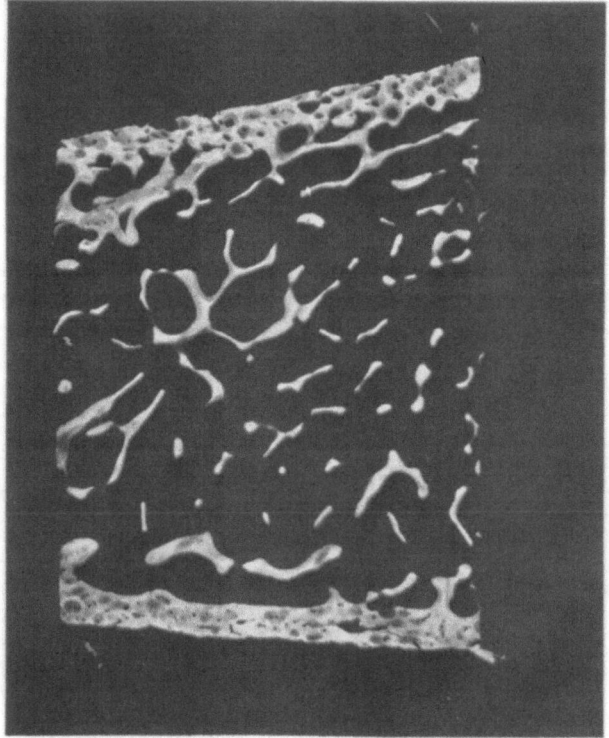

FIGURE 30. A microradiograph of a transilial bone biopsy as in Figure 26d. Both cortices and trabecular bone are intact (magnification ×7).

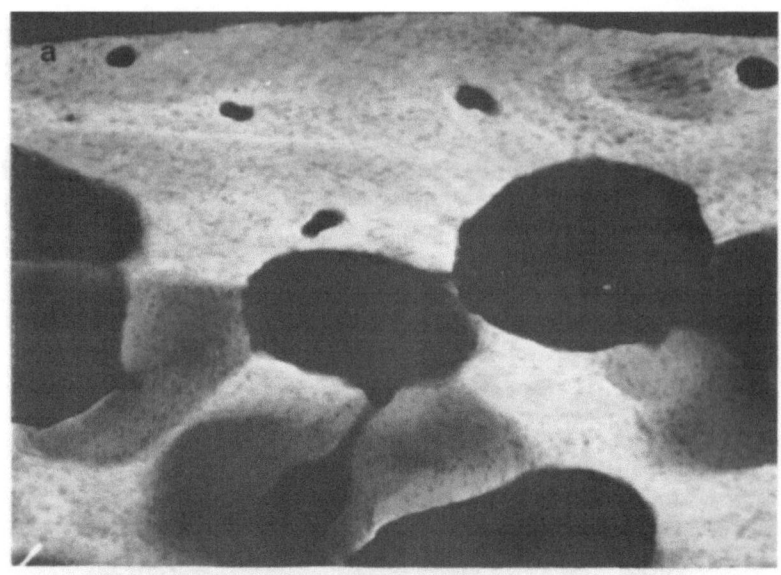

FIGURE 31a

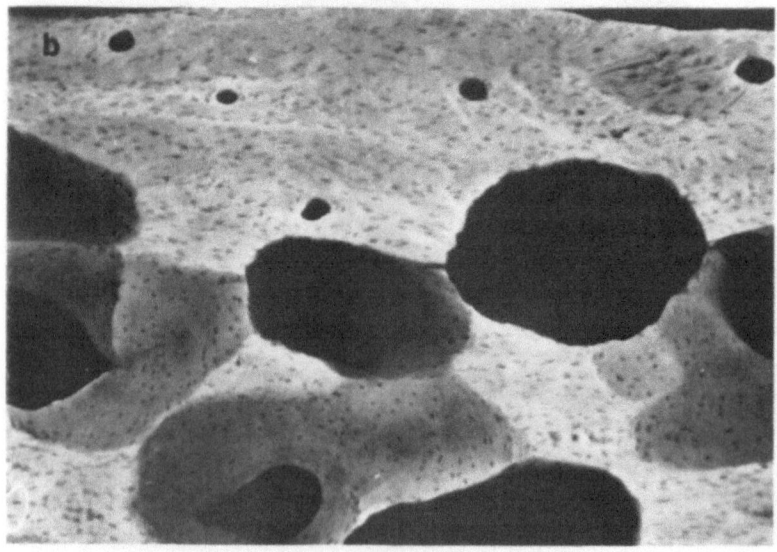

FIGURE 31b

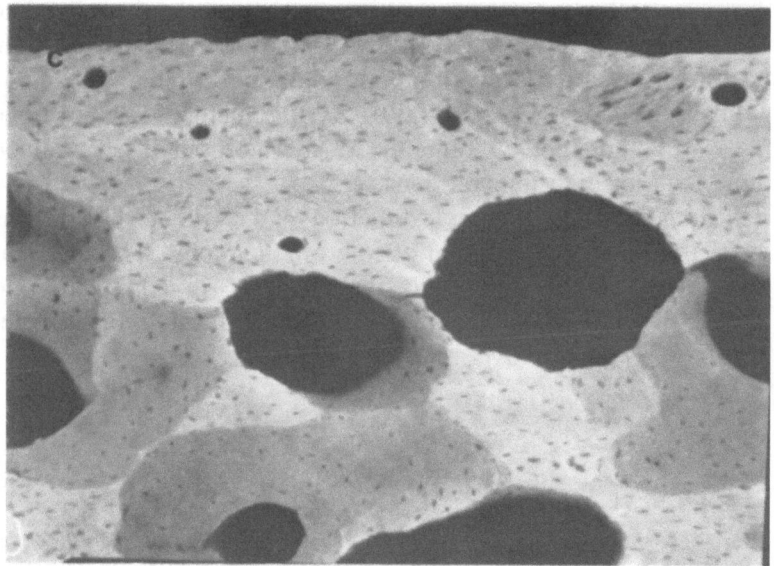

FIGURE 31c

FIGURE 31. Microradiographs of human cortical bone. (a) A 200 μm thick section; (b) the section ground down to 100 μm; and (c) the section further ground to 50 μm (magnification x 100).

μm in thickness (Jowsey *et al.*, 1965). Thicker sections tend to result in confusion because of overlying anatomical structures, while thinner sections decrease the difference between areas of bone of different mineral density (Figures 31a, b, and c). It is important to have sections of uniform and consistent thickness because of bone density and porosity measurements; any variation in the section thickness will be reflected in an increase or decrease in bone mass dependent on the thickness of the section rather than on real changes in density. Differences in mineralization of bone are the most obvious information to be derived from a microradiograph, the variations appearing as gradations of grayness and corresponding to areas of bone formed at different times. Such information cannot be derived from any other sort of preparation, such as a demineralized or mineralized section where differences in mineral density are not visible. The partial exception is the staining of mineralized bone with basic fuchsin (Frost, 1959). By this method areas of bone that are incompletely mineralized are more intensely stained than bone of high mineral density.

Quantitation of bone formation and bone resorption has been the major contribution of microradiography. The microradiograph and the stained section are used in conjunction to derive this information, and the method is most frequently referred to as quantitative microradiography.

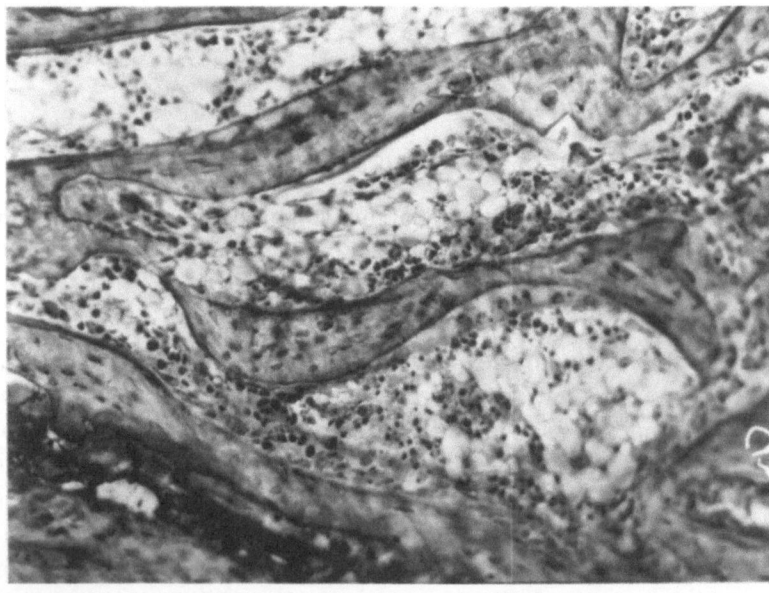

FIGURE 32. A stained, mineralized section of the metaphyseal area of a growing animal. The material is fixed in neutral formalin, embedded in methyl methacrylate, and stained with the Paragon stain (C and C Paragon Co., Inc., 190 Willow Avenue, Bronx, New York, 10454). The cell detail is good and the section is not broken or disrupted (magnification × 250).

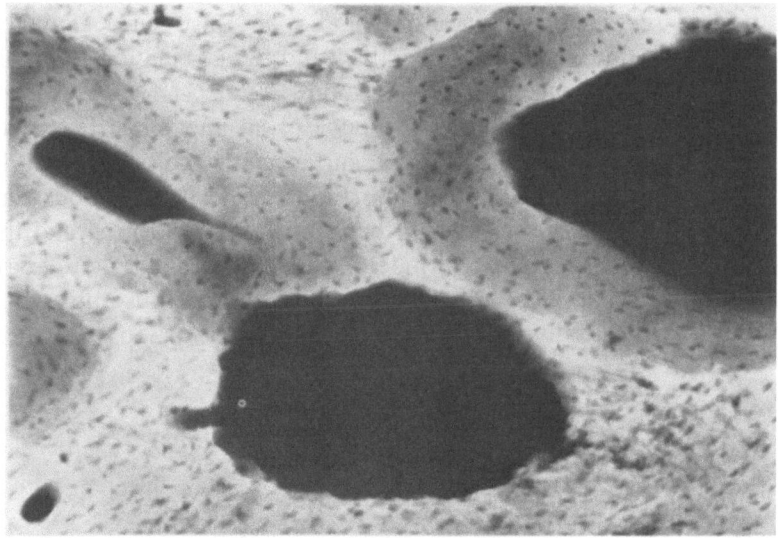

FIGURE 33. Microradiograph of cortical bone from a human being. A resorption cavity is seen in the lower center of the picture; active resorption is only occurring on part of the surface (magnification ×125).

After the microradiographs are made, the sections are ground to 40 μm in thickness and stained with the Paragon stain. Cell detail is excellent in such a preparation if the fixation and embedding is good (Figure 32). The major advantage is that the stained section can then be compared with the microradiograph and correlated with the more conventional bone formation and resorption parameters such as osteoblasts and tetracycline or osteoclasts. Bone formation, in a microradiograph, appears as a border of low density bone in which the lamellae are parallel to the surface. The density increases rapidly toward the soft-tissue space, either the Haversian canal, the bone marrow, or the periosteum, and there is no clear distinction between the least mineralized bone and the total blackness of the soft-tissue area (Figure 33). Such surfaces are covered with osteoid tissue and with a layer of cuboidal osteoblasts when compared with the stained section of the same area. They are also surfaces which have a double band of tetracycline, and the correlation with this evaluation of bone formation is good (Figure 34). Bone resorption is characterized by the presence of an uneven surface with bone lamellae at an angle to the surface, and the bone is nearly always of high mineral density (Figure 33). It is obvious that there should be a relationship between bone resorption and the number of osteoclasts, and indeed, this is the case (Figure 35a). There is also a close relationship between bone resorption and the serum parathyroid hormone levels (Figure 35b). Because

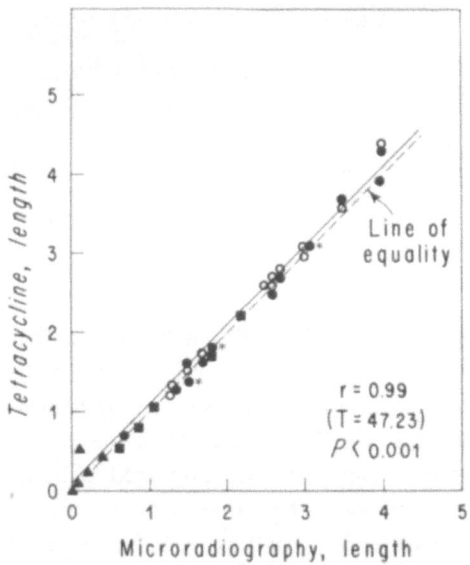

FIGURE 34. Relationship between bone formation evaluated by tetracycline uptake and by quantitative microradiography; 39 bone specimens, including 28 iliac crest biopsies from normal and abnormal human beings have been compared and the relationship is good. From Jowsey, 1973b. o = growing animals (11), • = normal humans (12), ■ = osteoporotic humans (11), ▲ = steroid-treated humans (5). Double label (* single label).

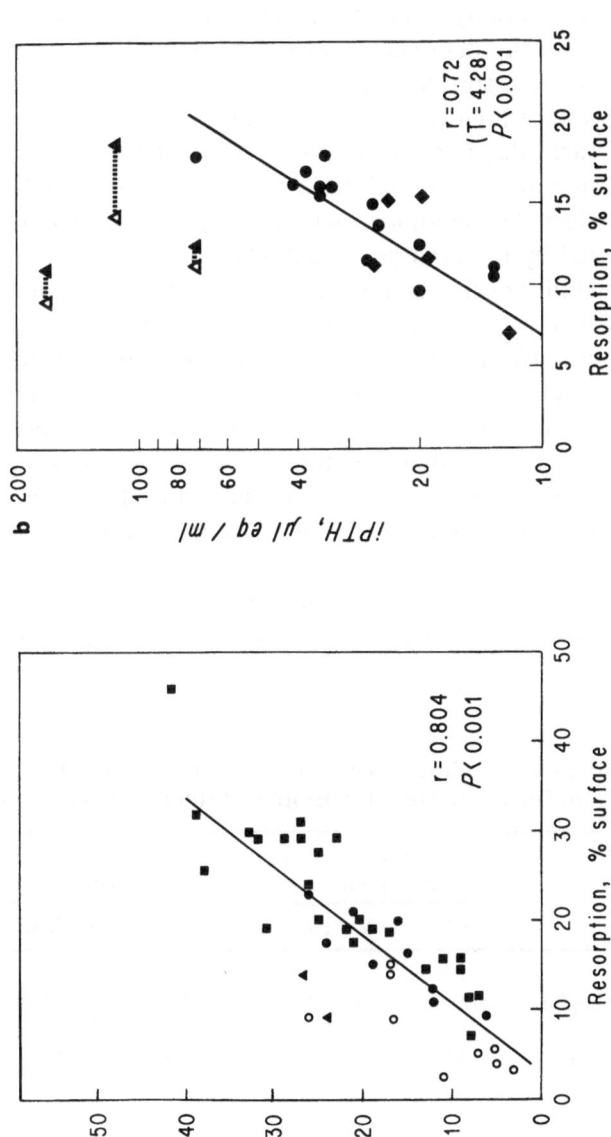

FIGURES 35a and b. Relationship between bone resorption measured by quantitative microradiography and (a) the number of osteoclasts present in the stained section (from Jowsey, 1973b) and (b) the serum immunoreactive parathyroid hormone in the patients at the time the biopsy was taken. (a): o = normal, • = osteoporotic, ■ = 2° hyperparathyroidism, ▲ = 1° hyperparathyroidism, ◆ = osteogenesis imperfecta. (b) • = osteoporosis, ▲ = 1° hyperparathyroidism.

Bordier reported a close correlation between the number of osteoclasts and serum parathyroid hormone (Bordier *et al.*, 1973a)
and also because of the data shown in Figure 35b, it is firmly
established that bone resorption measured by microradiography
represents both the cellular and the hormonal attributes of bone
resorption. In fact, the bone resorption values derived from
quantitative microradiography and the osteoclast numbers could
be used to validate the biological activity of parathyroid hormone as measured by immunoassay methods.

The repeatability of the data is good for both formation and
resorption and well within the variations seen in any ten year
age group (Figure 36). The interobserver error and error of the
method is low (Table 9). There is no doubt that some of the
high degree of accuracy comes from the size of the biopsy since
repeatability using a 5 mm diameter trephine was poor, and for
this reason the smaller biopsy was not considered useful except
for the diagnosis of such bone disorders as Paget's disease of
bone or chronic osteomalacia. Bone disorders or alterations in
bone turnover on the whole require quantitative evaluation of
formation, resorption, osteoid width, etc., and this is only accu-

TABLE 9. Errors in the Method of Quantitative Microradiography
Using a 8.0 mm Diameter Trephine Biopsy of the Iliac Crest

	Bone resorption		Bone formation	
	r [a]	Variance	r	Variance
Interobserver error				
(analysis by 2 people)	0.986	0.125	0.979	0.160
Site variation				
(biopsies 1 in. apart)	0.873	0.821	0.824	0.766
Section variation				
(different sections in				
the same biopsy)	0.885	1.114	0.844	0.650

[a] Correlation coefficient.

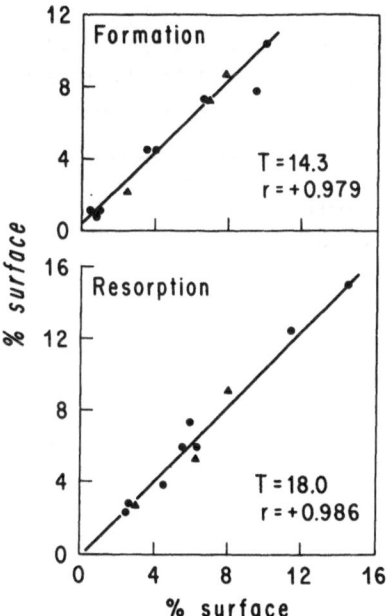

FIGURE 36. Repeatability in 11 iliac crest bone biopsies in normal human beings; resorption and formation are evaluated by quantitative microradiography and expressed as the percentage of the total surface in the biopsy (type Fig. 26d).

rate if a large enough area is analyzed. As previously mentioned, it is also essential that both cortical and trabecular bone be evaluated in order to obtain a realistic estimate of the metabolic state of the skeleton.

A problem that has already been mentioned is the relationship between the results in a biopsy and the general metabolism of the whole skeleton. Some idea of the representativeness of the results from a single biopsy can be obtained by comparing the results of the same analysis in different sites of the skeleton. This is carried out by analyzing formation and resorption in different sites in samples from the same individual (Table

TABLE 10. Correlation of Bone Turnover in Different
Skeletal Sites: Measurements of Bone Formation
and Resorption by Quantitative Microradiography

	r	t	p	Variance
Femur cortex vs. vertebra	0.843	4.435	<.001	5.204
Anterior iliac crest vs. vertebra	0.398	1.737	<.05	4.045
Posterior iliac crest vs. anterior iliac crest	0.822	9.132	<.001	1.388
Right anterior iliac crest vs. left anterior iliac crest	0.912	14.447	<.001	1.121

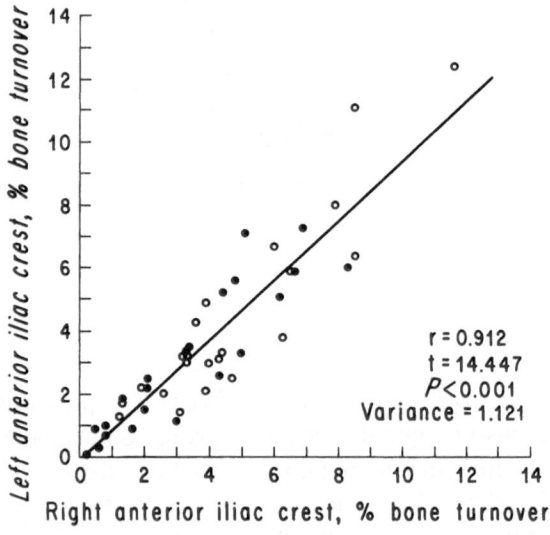

FIGURE 37. Bone turnover in different skeletal sites. Relationship
between bone formation and resorption measured by quantitative
microradiography in the left and right iliac crest of 23 individuals
with and without bone disease. The correlation is good and allows
a comparison to be made between left and right iliac crest biopsies
at different times. ● = formation, ○ = resorption.

10). The relationship between the different sites is poor, although the correlation is significant. Of primary importance is the repeatability between two similar sites that are to be compared at different times. For example, biopsies from the left and right anterior iliac crest have been used before and after various treatment regimes, and it is essential therefore that in the control state these two sites should be almost identical, in terms of bone cell activity, which appears to be so (Figure 37).

Chapter 5

Methods of Analysis

The majority of investigators interested in carrying out quantitation of bone biopsies count the cells within a certain area using a grid. The grid is placed in the eyepiece of the microscope and is projected onto the field at a magnification of about 100 times. The grid may be a series of points on a number of lines or it may consist of a cross-hatched area or merely an array of lines. If the grid is cross-hatched or if lines with points are used, it is most common to evaluate the event that is occurring at the grid intersections or at the point where the line crosses the bone surface to be analyzed. In a bone biopsy the presence of an osteoblast, of an osteoclast, or of an inactive surface are the three major events recorded. If enough events or hits are recorded to provide statistically valid results, the average number of events as a percentage of the total number of points is representative of the area of active cells as a fraction of the total area of the sample, which in turn reflects the section. Courpron, Merz, Bordier, Schultz, Sedlin, Teitelbaum, and Sherrard all utilize grids and point-count methods for evaluation of bone turnover (Courpron *et al.*, 1974; Merz and Schenk, 1970; Bordier *et al.*, 1964; Schultz and Delling, 1976a; Sedlin *et al.*, 1963; Sherrard *et al.*, 1974 and Teitelbaum *et al.*, 1976a). The exception is Jowsey who evaluates what is occurring on all of the surface rather than a finite number of randomly selected samples of the surface (see below).

The conversion of a measurement of length of surface or of area to one of three dimensions, thus permitting the section to reflect the biopsy, requires only that the section be infinitely thin with respect to the bone cells. Since sections are usually 10 μm in thickness, or thereabouts, and the bone cells are larger, the requirement is satisfied for bone formation and resorption. It is also satisfied for osteocytes since these cells, although only 10 by 15 μm in dimension, are generally over 50 μm from each other, and there will be no change in number unless the sections approach 50 μm in thickness or more. The most serious complication arises when bone volume determinations are made on sections of different thickness, and this will be discussed under the heading of porosity and volume analyses.

If the bone surface is analyzed where a line intersects with a surface, the values remain in terms of bone surface rather than volume; the section thickness must be infinitely small in this instance also, if the data are to be extrapolated from a section to a volume of bone. An alternative technique can be used and is frequently the method used in analyzing microradiographs; the method involves a photographic enlargement of the microradiograph and analysis of the entire surface of the microradiograph and corresponding section in one to three sections. This method is particularly useful when a limited number of sections are available; it can also be considered merely as an alternative to making numerous measurements on many sections. In the point-count method, using a grid, the section is viewed using a microscope and the data are recorded directly; in the photographic method, the section and microradiograph are also viewed with the aid of a microscope, the appearance is recorded on the photograph using colored lines (and thus establishing a permanent record of the bone surface activity), the length of these lines is measured with a perimeter (a small-toothed wheel with a handle that records the length of the line along which it is run), and the values are corrected for magnification. The results are usually

TABLE 11. Quantitation of Bone Turnover

Length of resorption surfaces	$=R$ (cm)
Length of formation surfaces	$=F$ (cm)
Length of inactive surfaces	$=I$ (cm)

$\therefore$ Total surface $= R + F + I$ (cm)

$\therefore$ percentage of bone resorption $= \dfrac{R}{R+F+I} \times 100$

$\therefore$ percentage of bone formation $= \dfrac{F}{R+F+I} \times 100$

expressed as a percentage of the total surface that is resorbing, forming, or inactive (Table 11). Surfaces covered by inactive osteoid can also be included in such an evaluation, as well as surfaces covered with active osteoid tissue.

There are two limitations of bone morphometric techniques which are inherent in any analysis of tissue. Assuming that the iliac crest biopsy is representative of bone turnover in the skeleton, the analysis of formation and resorption assumes that the cell counts represent, quantitatively, matrix deposition and bone removal. This limitation is concerned with the restriction of surface measurements when compared with measurements of rate. Bone turnover is three dimensional and bone resorption and formation, although conventionally viewed in cross section in two dimensions, is proceeding in a third dimension at a rate that will be reflected in the frequency with these events are seen in two dimensions. Any new site of resorption and formation or increase or decrease in the number of new sites will also be expressed in changes in the two-dimensional appearance. The radial rate at which resorption and formation are occurring, however, can only be measured for formation using multiple tetracycline bands. The radial rate of resorption is essentially impossible to measure in humans, even under the best of all possible circumstances; therefore, only the activity of bone surfaces can be quantitated and the extrapolation of such measurements to rates of bone formation and resorption have to be assumed to be constantly related to percentage surface values.

A constant relationship does not necessarily infer an identical one. Double tetracycline labeling techniques have allowed accurate measurements of the rate of bone matrix deposition that appears to be progressing at about 1 μm per day (Frost, 1960; Lee *et al.*, 1965). In children and in Paget's disease of bone this value is somewhat higher, while in immobilization the rate appears to be decreased. The variations in rate, however, are small compared with the changes that occur in the percentage of surface undergoing formation.

Bone resorption appears to be occurring not only over a larger surface than that occupied by the osteoclast itself, but also at a faster rate than osteoblastic bone formation. As already mentioned, it is essentially impossible to measure bone resorption rates in bone from human beings. In adult dogs both resorption and formation rates are measurable by using tetracycline labeling techniques and longitudinal sections of remodeling cortical bone (Jaworski and Lok, 1972). The longitudinal rate of formation and resorption are similar; however, the radial rate of resorption appears to occur about four times more rapidly than the radial rate of formation (Table 12). Therefore, by assuming

TABLE 12

Radial	Longitudinal
Resorption rate in dogs (μm/day)	
7.1 ± (SD 2.9)	39.2 ± (SD 13.7)[a]
9.2 ± (SE 0.5)	43.6 ± (SE 1.0)[b]
Formation rate in dogs (μm/day)	
2.0 ± (SD 0.3)[c]	44.4 ± (SD 12.0)[a]
1.4 ± (SD 0.1)[c]	43.6 ± (SE 0.7)[b]

[a] Jaworski and Lok, 1972.
[b] Jaworski *et al.*, 1975.
[c] Lee *et al.*, 1965.

a similar rate of bone resorption and formation, the amount of bone removed is underestimated. This is possibly the explanation of some of the discrepancies which arise when bone cell counts per unit surface are used to evaluate bone turnover. Such measurements may result in values for formation that are greater than those for resorption (Wakamatsu and Sissons, 1969; Sherrard *et al.*, 1974) when it is established beyond doubt that bone loss is occurring, as with increasing age and in osteoporosis. Methods evaluating bone formation using osteoid surface, tetracycline, or quantitative microradiography should and do correspond accurately with the length of surface covered with osteoblasts. However, the length of surface occupied by bone resorption is generally greater than that covered by osteoclasts for reasons described above (Owen, 1971), and even this is an underestimate if the radial rate, which cannot be evaluated by either cellular or by surface measurements, is not taken into account.

METHODS OF ANALYSIS

Chapter 6

Identification of
Bone Cell Activity

Ultimately the validity of any of the methods of quantitative bone morphology depend on accurate identification of the bone cell activity. The cells and structures that are evaluated vary from one investigator to another, but they nearly always include bone formation which is distinguished either by osteoblasts, by osteoid covered by osteoblasts, by the presence of low density bone in a microradiograph, or by a double (or less satisfactorily, a single) tetracycline band. The active osteoblasts involved in new matrix deposition are generally cuboidal and lined up in sheets on the bone surface and are relatively easy to recognize (Figure 38). They are invariably associated with unmineralized osteoid tissue, with tetracycline uptake and, except in osteomalacia, with a mineralization front. Measurements of the length of surface covered by osteoid tissue which is covered with a layer or sheet of osteoblasts, often termed active osteoid, can also be used rather than a count of osteoblasts. The osteoid tissue can be seen most readily in undemineralized, unstained sections where it appears as a translucent layer containing osteocytes (Figure 39). A double label of tetracycline, resulting from two or more injections of tetracycline, given at an interval

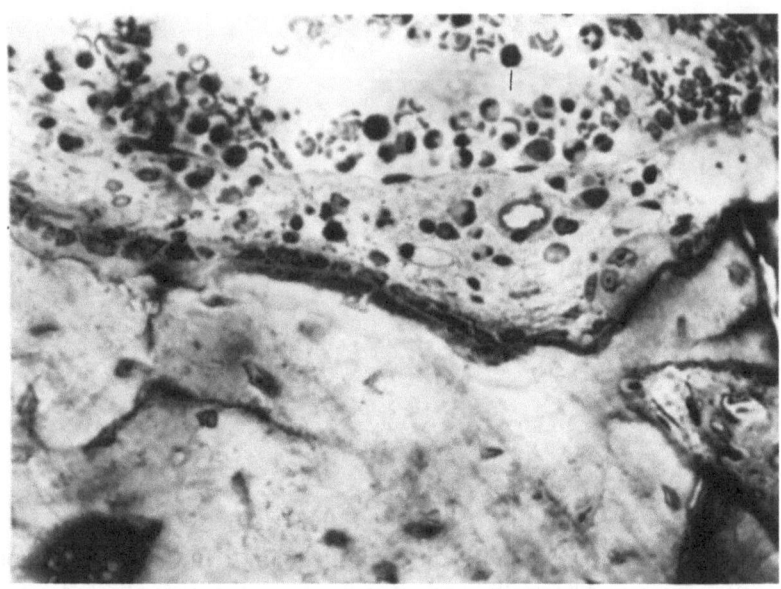

FIGURE 38. A stained, mineralized section with a layer of osteoblasts on the bone surface with a narrow band of osteoid beneath. To the right is an osteoclast (magnification × 640).

of a few days, also produces evidence of new matrix production
and is probably the most certain method to evaluate the presence
of new bone deposition (Figure 40). However, so many patients
and animals have received previous doses of tetracycline that
the majority of biopsy samples are labeled many times before
the intended two labels are administered, and it is often difficult
to distinguish the previous labels from those given for the purpose of measuring bone formation.

Osteoblast cell counts correlate well with other parameters
of bone formation, such as osteoid and tetracycline. Schenk
found a correlation of 0.948 between osteoblasts evaluated in
terms of cell area (mm ^{2} osteoblasts/cm ^{3}) per unit volume of section and osteoid volume per unit volume of bone (Schenk *et al.,*

1973). If microradiography is the technique being used, the length of the band of low density bone is measured (Figure 41a), microradiographic evaluation of bone formation correlates well with tetracycline uptake ($r = 0.99$, $t = 47.2$), and the variance is small (Table 13). Osteoblasts, osteoid, and tetracycline evaluation of bone formation have all been measured using the point-counting grid method, while osteoid, tetracycline, and microradiographic evidence of bone formation have been measured photographically, with the total surfaces being evaluated.

When bone formation ceases, the osteoblasts become flattened and less cuboidal and may still be associated with osteoid.

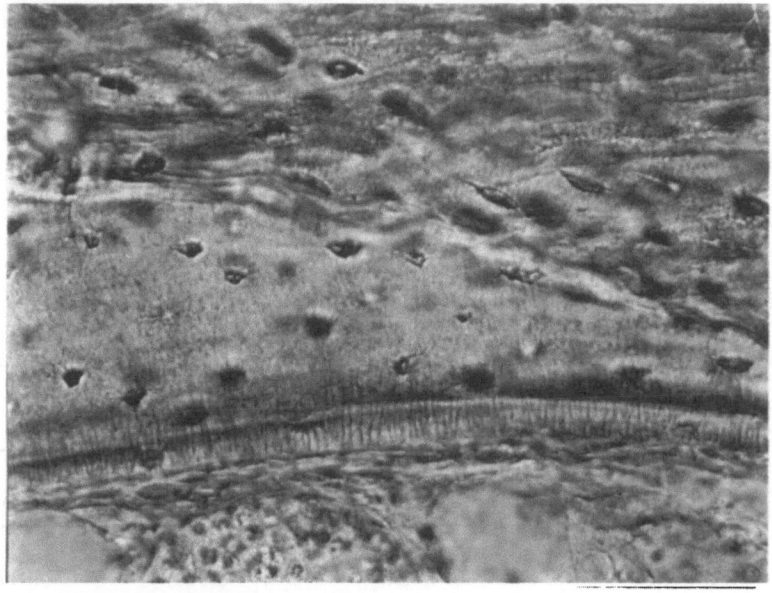

FIGURE 39. An unstained, mineralized bone section, showing a border of unmineralized bone, or osteoid, with osteocytes and canaliculi. The osteoid border is covered by a layer of osteoblasts (magnification ×400).

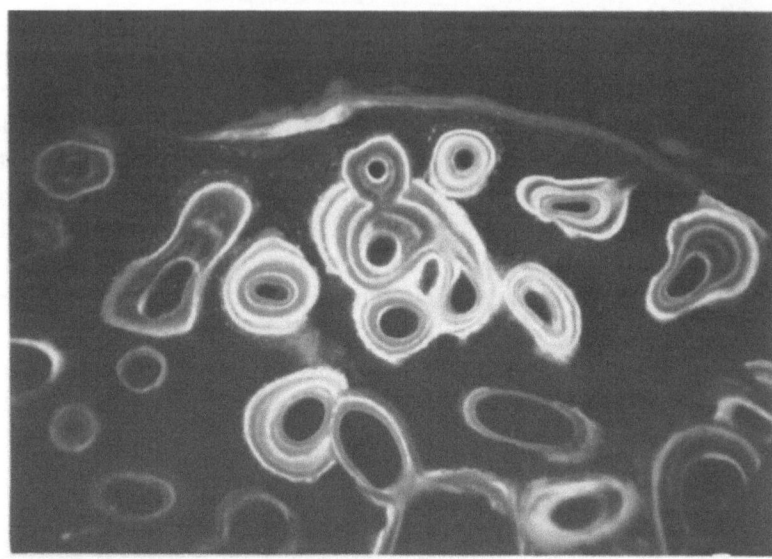

FIGURE 40. Repeated injections of tetracycline in an adult dog to show the bands of fluorescence which correspond to the injections. The dark bands between correspond to the period between injections during which bone has continued to be laid down (magnification × 50).

TABLE 13. Relationships between Different Parameters of Bone Formation and Resorption Evaluated by Quantitative Microradiography

Parameter	Number of observations	Correlation coefficient (r)	Variance
Tetracycline and formation	34	0.993	0.017
iPTH and resorption	19	0.720	1.58
Osteoclast number per unit area and resorption	45	0.804	3.24

Whether they still produce matrix is questionable, and there is no doubt that fixation and staining procedures may often produce a shrunken-looking cell in place of what *in vivo* was cuboidal and plump. However, inactive bone surfaces with no osteoid layer are lined by sparse connective tissue cells. These cells, with the osteoblasts and osteoclasts, may form the bone membrane which separates the bone tissue from the extracellular, extravascular fluid. There is every reason to believe that a physiological or anatomical membrane is present that allows the composition of bone fluid to be different from the composition of the surrounding medium. *In vivo*, it is likely that the cy-

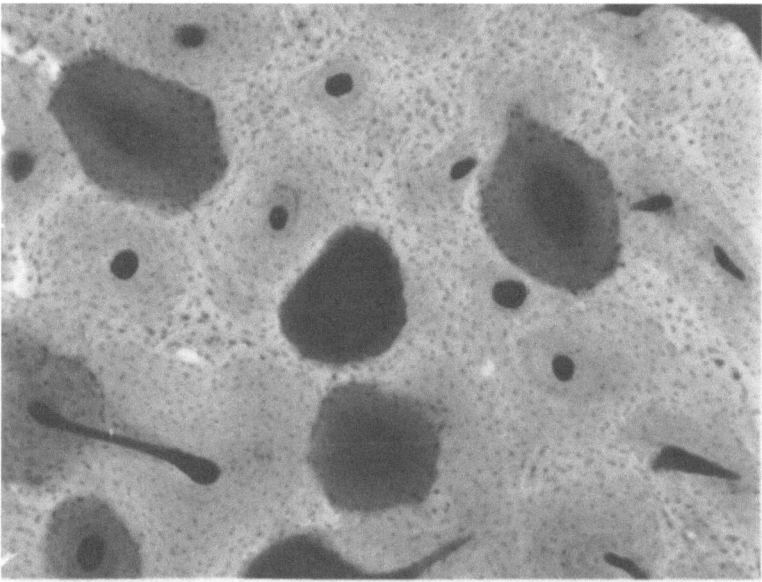

FIGURE 41a. A microradiograph of a cross section of human cortical bone. The recently formed osteones are incompletely mineralized and therefore appear dark on the microradiograph. The length of the inner perimeter of the Haversian systems is the length of surface undergoing bone formation (magnification × 125).

toplasm of the cells covering the bone surface is spread out over a large surface and abuts onto cytoplasmic extensions of adjacent cells, thus forming an anatomical membrane. The dedifferentiated osteoblasts or mesenchyme cells possibly fulfill this function on the inert surfaces of bone.

Flattened osteoblasts are easily distinguished from the plump cuboidal cells that are present in areas of active matrix formation; also, the characteristic bone-forming surface seen in a microradiograph appears of low density but with a sclerotic border when formation ceases (Figure 41b). Inactive osteoid, that is, osteoid that is no longer in the process of formation, may be more difficult to differentiate from osteoid that is being

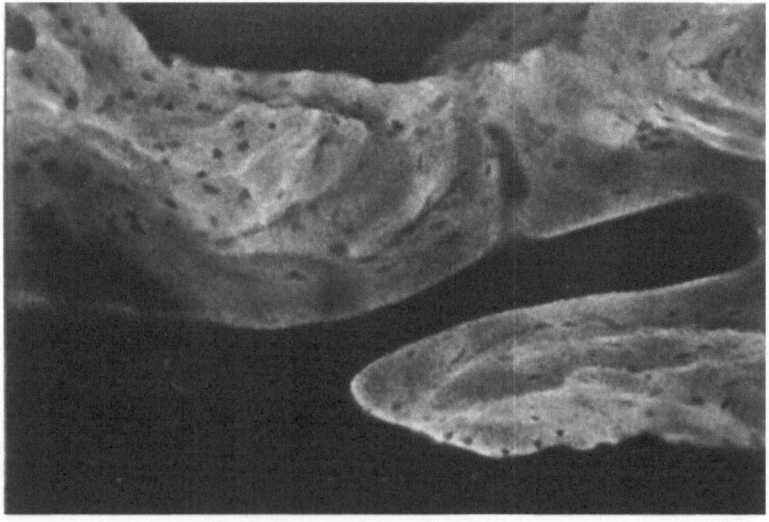

FIGURE 41b. A microradiograph of a cross section of human cortical bone. An area of low mineral density is bordered by a narrow line of sclerosis indicating cessation of recent bone formation (magnification × 250).

TABLE 14a. Bone Formation Surfaces in Normal Adult Individuals

Investigator	Year	Percentage (mean)
Bordier *et al.*	1973b	4.5 ± 2 SD 4.0 [a]
Schulz and Delling	1976b	2.0 [a]
Jowsey *et al.*	1965	2.6 ± 1 SD 1.2 [b]
Jowsey	1977b	3.2 ± 1 SD 2.7 [b]
Schenk *et al.*	1973	4.3 ± 1 SD 3.4 [a]
Schenk	1976	4.5 ± 1 SD 3.9 [a]
Sherrard *et al.*	1973	16.9 ± 1 SD 7.2 [a]
Sherrard *et al.*	1974	17.7 ± 1 SD 8.5 [a]
Wakamatsu and Sissons	1969	6.3 [a]

[a] Percentage of trabecular surface covered with osteoblasts or osteoid.
[b] Percentage of cortical and trabecular surface undergoing formation evaluated by quantitative microradiography.

actively deposited, and this may explain the high "formation" figures in reports where this method is used (Table 14a).

Bone formation measured by the presence of osteoblasts, by double tetracycline label, or by quantitative microradiography has clearly defined parameters in bone sections. The differences that are reported by different investigators are largely the result of different sites of the sample that are anlyzed, although they are generally derived from iliac crest biopsies. With the exception of the consistently high values reported by Sherrard and co-workers (Sherrard *et al.*, 1974), in studies in which osteoid tissue was used to identify bone formation, the majority of methods report values of about 3 or 4% as being the average value in normal adults (Table 14a).

Bone resorption carried out by osteoclasts results in indentations on the bone surface, the Howship's lacunae (Figure 42). By the point-counting method the percentage of bone surface occupied by the osteoclasts or by Howship's lacunae containing osteoclasts gives an estimate of the activity of bone resorption. The photographic method gives a similar measure of resorption, the extent of the surface evaluated merely being much greater,

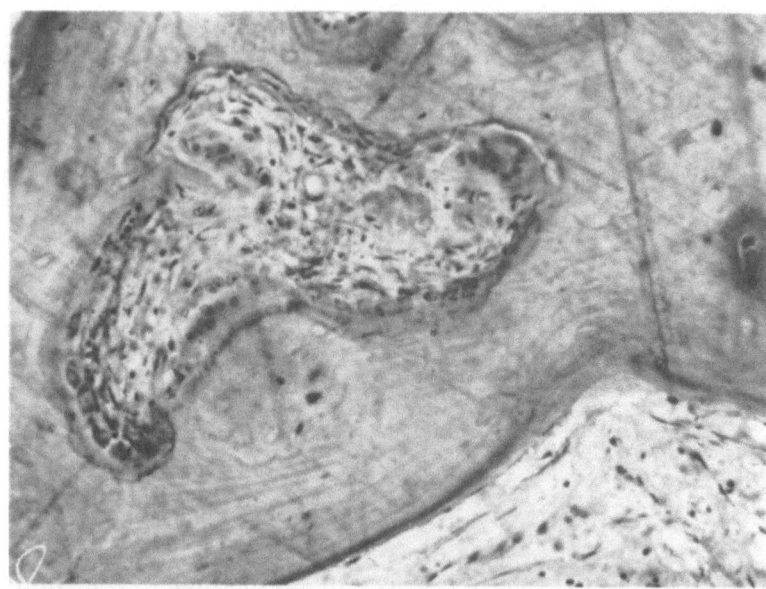

FIGURE 42. A stained, mineralized section of human cortical bone showing a resorption cavity with multinucleate osteoclasts and two areas of new bone formation. The osteoclasts are lying in the scalloped indentations, the Howship's lacunae (magnification × 250).

and irregular, crenated surfaces indicate bone resorption. In a histological, stained section the surface appears deeply stained, while in a microradiograph the surface is uneven and generally well mineralized (Figure 43). The osteoclasts appear to be surrounded by a large area where bone resorption is occurring that includes a greater percentage of the bone surface than that covered by the cell when observed in a fixed, dehydrated, and stained section. Autoradiographic techniques have shown that in a 9-h period almost twice the length of surface actually covered by an osteoclast is being resorbed (Owen and Shetlar, 1968). Since electron microscope pictures have suggested that the resorptive activity of the osteoclast is limited by the clear zone that

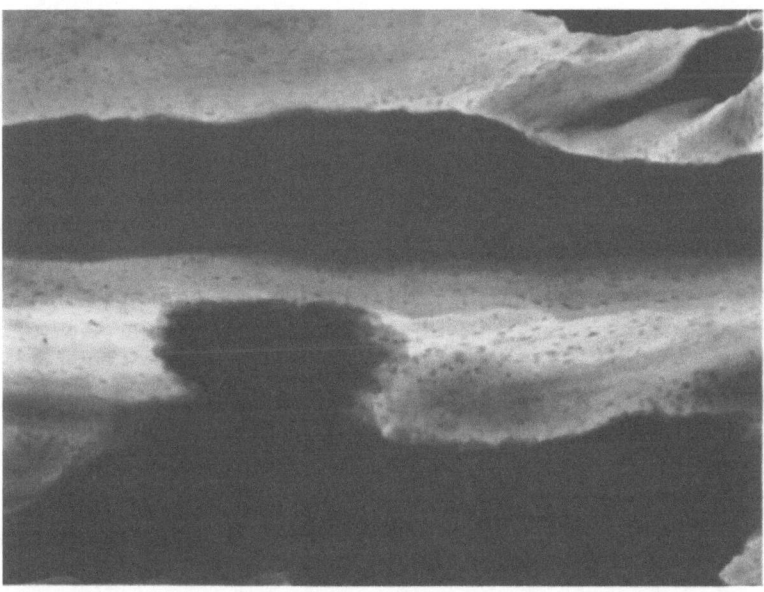

FIGURE 43. Microradiograph of cortical bone from a human being. Most of the bone is non-Haversian lamellar bone and a small resorption cavity lies in the center of the picture (magnification ×125).

occupies the perimeter of the cell, it is likely that the process of fixation and dehydration shrinks the cell to smaller dimensions than those that occur *in vivo*. For this reason, osteoclastic resorption, as estimated by cell counts, is likely to be an underestimate of the activity of the resorbing process. The relationship between bone resorption evaluated by counting osteoclasts and by parathyroid hormone levels is close (Figure 35b) (Table 13).

Bone resorption measurements by various investigators appear to be more variable, as is true for formation values, partly because of the difference in the sample of bone analyzed (Table 14b). Samples containing only trabecular bone tend to be lower, although reports from the same individual are generally in agreement. The exception to the latter is Bordier who reported 10.4% in 1964 and 0.6% in 1973 as an average value for re-sorption, a difference explained by the earlier data being derived from measurements of Howship's lacunae rather than from osteoclast counts (Bordier *et al.*, 1964, 1973b).

Osteoid is now generally measured in undemineralized sections (Meyer, 1956). These are prepared by fixing the bone in formalin buffered at pH 7.2 to prevent any demineralization of the specimen, with the material embedded in celloidin or methacrylate and sections cut with a microtome, a circular saw, or a blade. Double embedding, involving placing the bone first in celloidin and then in wax, has also been used (Ball, 1957). The sections prepared and cut using a microtome frequently suffer from cracking as the hard section slides up the knife blade surface; this can be prevented by sticking tape onto the surface of the block before cutting the section and then removing the tape after sticking the section or sections on a microscope slide. Despite these precautions and certainly without them, the sections are frequently cracked and the cellular contents are pulled away from the bone surface if a knife is used, even if it is a heavy knife and motor driven (Figures 44 and 45). Superior

TABLE 14b. Bone Resorption Surfaces in Normal Adult Individuals

Investigator	Year	Percentage (mean)
Bordier *et al.*	1964	10.4 ± 1.7
Bordier *et al.*	1973b	0.6 ± 2 SD 1.0^a
Meunier *et al.*	1973b	3.2 ± 0.9^a
Wakamatsu and Sissons	1969	5.0^a
Schenk	1976	0.5^a
Sherrard *et al.*	1973	$4.9 \pm$ SD 3.3^a
Sherrard *et al.*	1974	$4.4 \pm$ SD 2.1^a
Jowsey	1977b	$4.9 \pm$ SD 2.6^b

[a] Percentage of trabecular surface covered with osteoclasts.
[b] Percentage of cortical and trabecular surface undergoing resorption evaluated by quantitative microradiography.

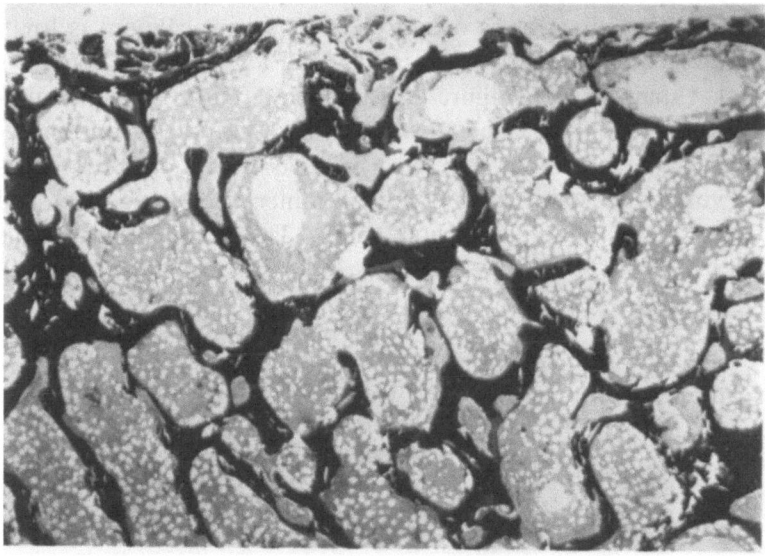

FIGURE 44. Stained, undecalcified section cut with a microtome. There are some rents and disruptions in trabeculae which have been produced by the knife (magnification × 16).

preparations are produced by methyl-methacrylate-embedded and sawn sections (Figure 46) (Jowsey *et al.*, 1965).

Osteoid can be easily recognized in an unstained section. It is translucent and lies on a bone surface and can be positively identified by the presence of canaliculi and osteocytes which are present within the osteoid (Figure 47). On the side between the osteoid and bone, a narrow band of granular material is normally present, the mineralization front. Mineralization occurs in a narrow band behind the osteoid, as a granular area, consisting of new foci of mineral (Figure 47). Normally approximately 15 days' worth of osteoid is laid down before mineralization occurs, and since osteoid is produced in an adult man at the rate of about 1 μm per day, normal osteoid is 15 μm thick. If for some reason mineralization is defective (i.e., serum calcium is low), then osteoid production continues and the osteoid border is thicker than normal (Figure 48). In such circumstances the mineralization front is absent, except in healing mineralization defects. Stained sections may also be used. The most common is the von Kossa stain which colors all mineralized bone black and leaves the unmineralized bone pink. The von Kossa stain is

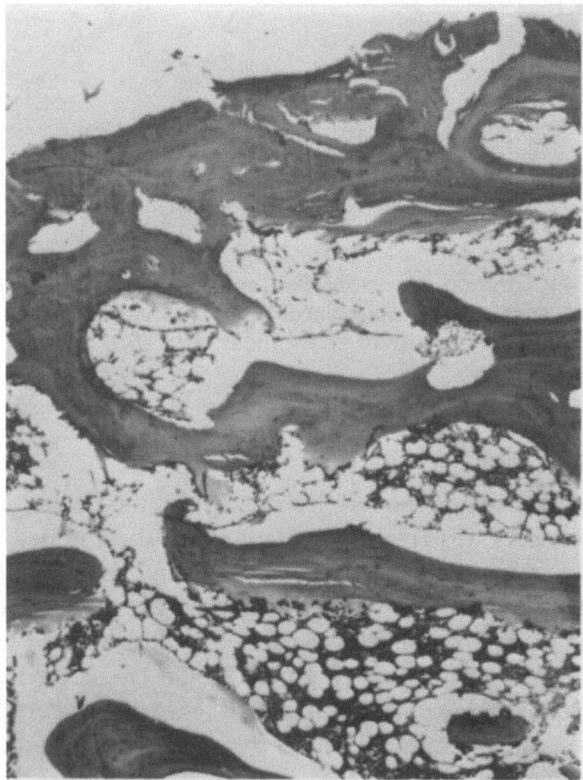

FIGURE 45. Stained, undemineralized section cut with a knife. The marrow has shrunk away or has been torn away from the bone surface, making evaluation of bone surface activity difficult (magnification ×64).

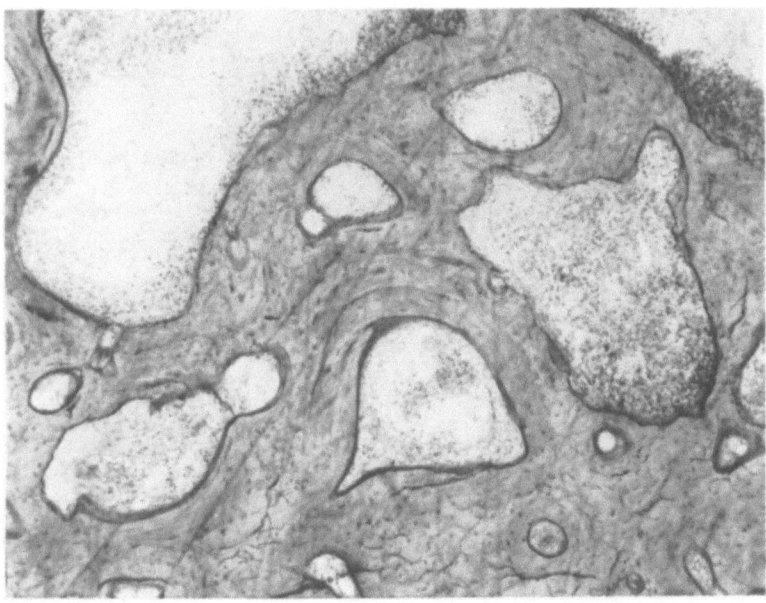

FIGURE 46. Stained, undecalcified section of bone cut with a circular saw. There is no break in the bone section and the soft tissue
has remained in contact with the bone surfaces (magnification
×64).

specific for phosphate and carbonate and therefore, in bone, can
be considered reasonably specific for calcium. Hematoxylin and
eosin can also be used since hematoxylin colors only the mineralized bone basophilically, even though the basophilia cannot be
considered specific for calcium. The stain is one conventionally
used in demineralized sections and if the material is only partially demineralized, then the distinction between osteoid and
bone (strictly speaking bone is osteoid *and* mineral) can be seen
(Figure 49). However, to be sure that osteoid is indeed unmineralized and does not represent artificial loss of mineral, an
undemineralized preparation is best, and the stain that is most commonly used is the Goldner stain in which the mineralized

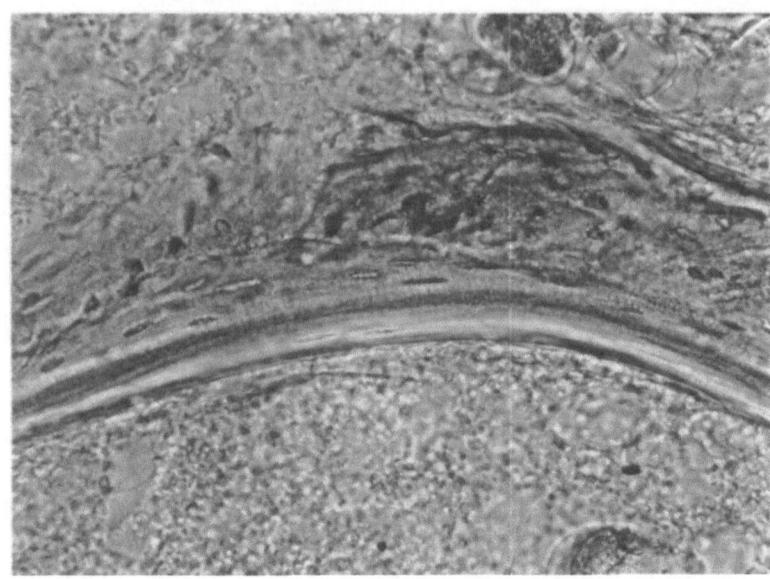

FIGURE 47. Active osteoid in an unstained mineralized section. There are osteocytes in the matrix and there is a mineralization front adjacent to the mineralized bone. Osteoblasts are just discernable on the marrow surface of the osteoid (magnification × 250).

bone is green, the osteoid is red, and the cells are red to brown. It takes a long time to stain a section (65 min) and involves 12 different steps. A shorter procedure, which results in pale pink bone, red osteoid, and pale red cells, is the Paragon stain which gives good cell detail and only involves 1 step and a 5-min time period (Figures 17, 21, and 32). Other stains have also been used (Meyer, 1956).

Prestaining of unmineralized osteoid appears to be an effective method which has the advantage that the bone can later be demineralized, embedded in paraffin, and cut by conventional methods (Yoshiki, 1973). Freshly removed bone is fixed in 0.5% cyanuric chloride in methanol containing 1% N-methyl morpholine. The cyanuric chloride reacts with the unmin-

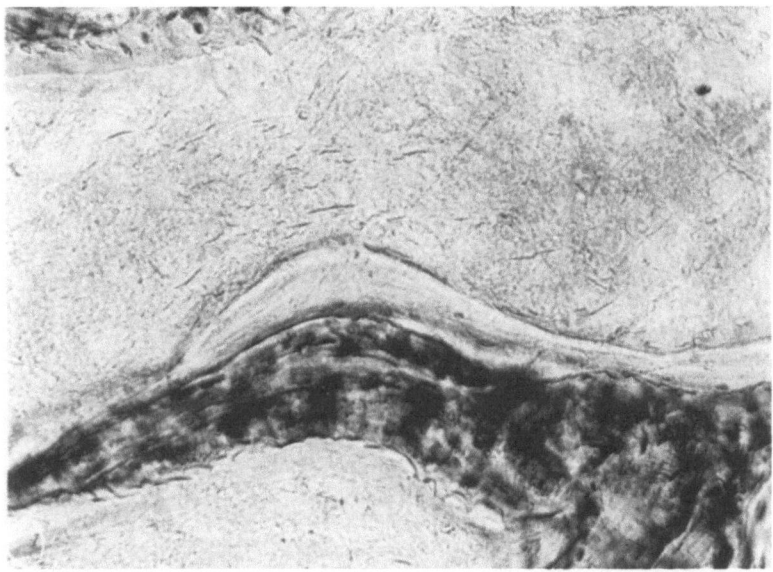

FIGURE 48. An unstained, mineralized bone section from a patient with osteomalacia. The dark bone spicule has a wide osteoid border on its upper surface that lacks a mineralization front (magnification × 200).

eralized osteoid while mineralized bone remains unstained. The bone tissue can be stained with hematoxylin and eosin or other connective tissue stains after demineralization in 10% EDTA.

The mention of demineralized sections brings up the alternative explanation of the presence of osteoid which is the theory of halisteresis. This theory was supported by von Recklinhausen (1910) and more recently by Bohatirchuk (1966). The theory suggested that the presence of osteoid represented mineralized bone from which the mineral had been removed. However, the almost invariable association of osteoid with osteoblasts and recently deposited mineral, visualized autoradiographically, indicates that osteoid is the first step in bone formation and never

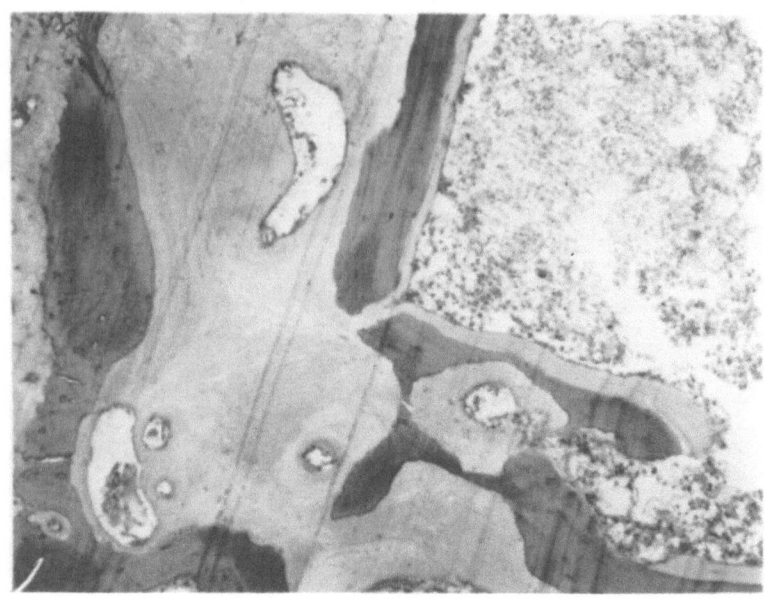

FIGURE 49. Cross section of stained, partially demineralized bone from a patient with osteomalacia. The dark areas represent bone containing mineral while the pale areas are of unmineralized matrix (magnification × 320).

has contained mineral. In addition, electron microscopic evidence points to a dissolution of collagen and mineral simultaneously in the process of bone resorption, and free mature crystals have never been observed in association with borders of collagen fibers of any significant size.

The successful recognition of osteoid tissue and the presence or absence of a mineralization front are two features of bone morphology that are quantitated to evaluate osteomalacia. The development of morphological osteomalacia occurs in four steps: (1) The absence of a mineralization front, which rapidly reflects a failure of mineralization; theoretically a lack of calcium or phosporus, both of which are necessary for mineralization of osteoid, should be seen as an absence of the granular line between the osteoid and bone within a day of the systemic defect. (2) After a few days, if mineralization fails to occur, continued osteoid formation will result in an increase in thickness of osteoid. (3) Bone formation in any one place only seems to occur for a certain time; Haversian systems and trabeculae are of a definite size (about 500 μm diameter for Haversian systems in adult man and 120 μm for trabeculae in adult man) (Jowsey, 1966). When osteoid deposition ceases there may be osteoid borders of 20 to 200 μm in width remaining. (4) The final step is in the accumulation of osteoid on a larger than normal number of surfaces. This occurs because new sites of bone formation arise and osteoid is laid down and remains unmineralized. It is usually at this stage of morphological osteomalacia that clinical symptoms and biochemical abnormalities are first seen. A large percent of the surface may eventually become encased in unmineralized osteoid and make the bone unavailable for its normal homeostatic function (Figure 50).

It is evident that the most sensitive and also the first sign of a mineralization defect is the lack of a calcification or mineralization front. An approximate measure of the presence or absence of a mineralization front is obtained from an undemineralized section. This should preferably be unstained, merely because a number of staining procedures involve a low pH solution which may remove the more labile mineral of the mineralization front. The percentage of the osteoid border occupied by the granular band is evaluated "by eye" in a significant number of areas or with an integrating eyepiece using the point-count method, and the data are averaged. In normal individuals 84.6% ($\pm$ SD 10%) of the osteoid has a mineralization front (Bordier et al., 1973b). In comparison, a group of patients with osteoporosis studied by the same investigators had a somewhat lower value for the mineralization front, $73 \pm 8.4\%$, and 6 out of 11 patients demonstrated values below one standard deviation of the normal mean. The data suggest that in this group of patients there was some defect in mineral metabolism that

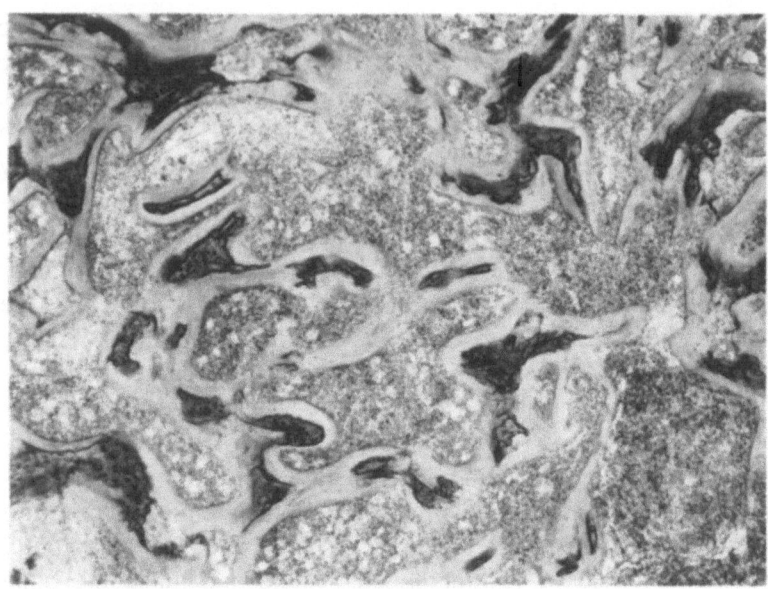

FIGURE 50. Stained section of mineralized bone from a patient with osteomalacia. The trabecular bone is almost entirely covered with unmineralized osteoid, making the mineralized bone "unavailable" for resorption by osteoclasts (magnification × 40).

tended to make them "osteomalacic," although not to a degree that was associated with the overt biochemical and symptomatic indications of the disease. Indeed, 4 out of 7 showed malabsorption, and 7 out of 11 demonstrated a total osteoid surface that was above one standard deviation from the normal mean, 6 being the same patients that showed a reduced mineralization front.

　　If an osteomalacic situation is corrected, the first evidence of bone healing will be the appearance of the mineralization front. The granular deposit may be patchy and is likely to be found throughout the osteoid border rather than in a narrow line adjacent to the mineralized bone. Mineralization generally continues until all the bone contains some mineral; however, the osteoid close to the vascular, soft-tissue surface will mineralize completely first, followed by the osteoid behind it, while patches of bone nearest the cement line or toward the center of a trabeculum may not mineralize (Figure 51) (Raina, 1973). The appearance in a mineralized unstained section is clear but not as obvious as the variation in mineral density seen in the microradiograph (Figure 52). Similarly, if there is a mineralization defect when bone is being laid down, the area around the osteocytes frequently remains incompletely mineralized (Figure 53). The appearance seen in Figures 51 and 52 is therefore characteristic of an adult-onset osteomalacia that is partially or completely healed, such as in an individual with malabsorption that

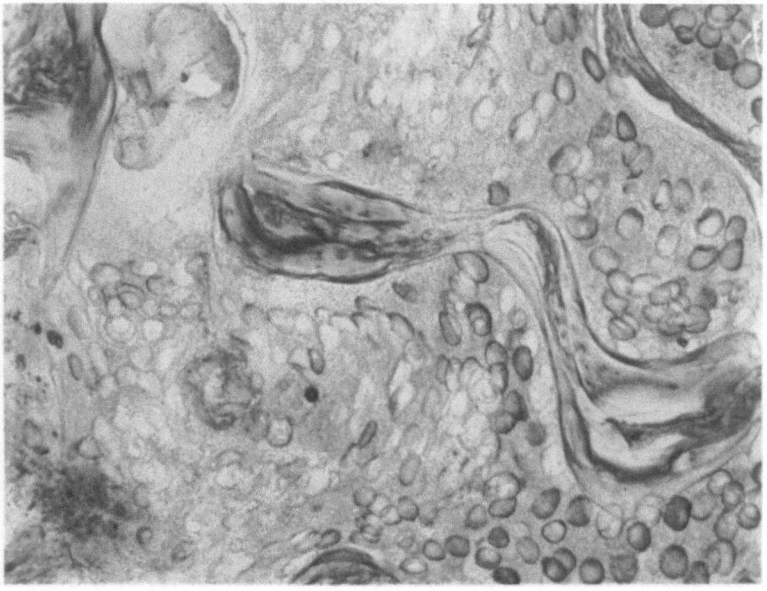

FIGURE 51. An unstained, mineralized section from a patient with chronic and active osteomalacia. The dark area represents poorly mineralized tissue; unmineralized osteoid covers the trabeculae (magnification × 64).

has been corrected, while the appearance in Figure 53 is a feature typical of hereditary forms of osteomalacia, such as vitamin-D-resistant rickets, although it will also occur when bone formation is taking place in the presence of a mineralization defect. Fluoride administration in the absence of adequate calcium will produce such an appearance (Figure 9d) since the fluoride stimulates bone formation while the inadequate calcium prevents normal bone mineralization. It may be that the poorly mineralized osteoid will remain permanently uncalcified as the result of some irreversible change in the matrix (Johnson,

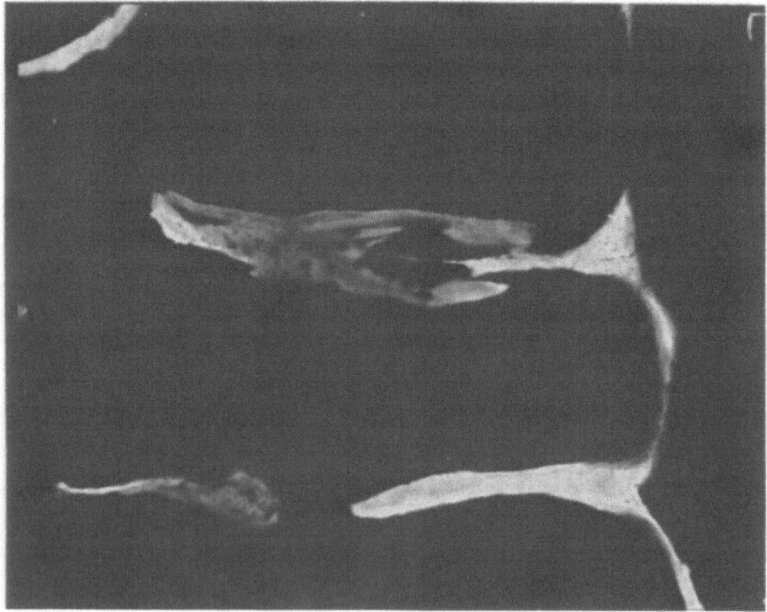

FIGURE 52. A microradiograph of trabecular bone from a patient with osteomalacia that has been successfully treated. The poorly mineralized bone lies in the center of the trabeculum, and bone of somewhat higher density covers it (magnification ×64).

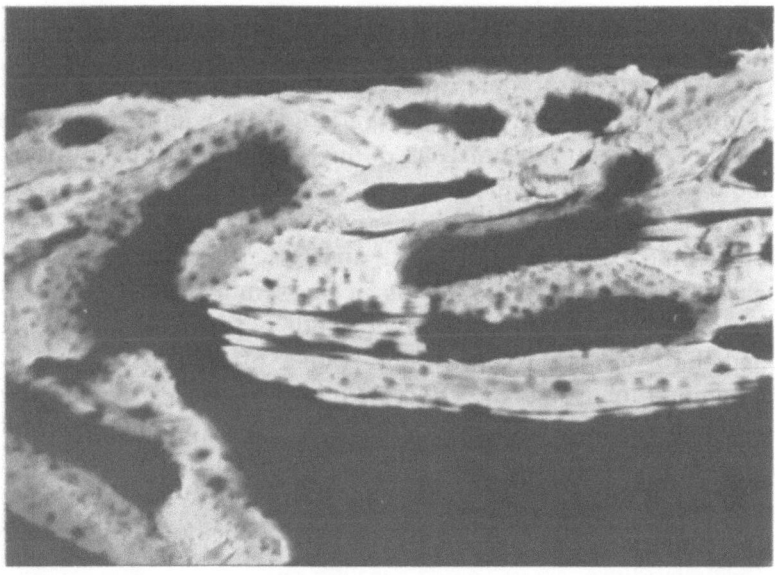

FIGURE 53. A microradiograph of a section of mineralized bone from a patient with vitamin-D-resistant rickets. Bone immediately around the osteocytes is poorly mineralized; unlike osteocytic osteolysis, the matrix is present in normal amounts, so the appearance on a demineralized specimen is normal (magnification × 64).

1964). Mineralization depends on an available supply of calcium and phosphorus; absence of sufficient amounts of either of these will prevent mineralization. Calcium in the serum can be reduced effectively by parathyroidectomy and occurs occasionally as a clinical syndrome as the result of a total parathyroidectomy or more rarely, in hypoparathyroidism. Lack of mineralization may also occur as a result of hypophosphatemia (Burkhart and Jowsey, 1966; Salassa *et al.*, 1970). Both conditions result in a failure of mineralization and a decrease in the mineralization front, followed by a widening of the unmineralized osteoid border and the morphological appearance of osteomalacia. The width of osteoid reported is almost always a mean value derived from a number of measurements made of the average width of a significant number of borders. Generally, 10 to 20 osteoid borders must be measured to achieve a meaningful value; the greater the variation in width, the larger number that must be measured. In normal individuals the osteoid width varies somewhat with age. In children, the average width is approximately 10 μm, a value that is lower than at any other time except in the elderly, and perhaps reflecting the high calcium and phosphorus levels in the serum that are found in children. The maximum normal width is found in the second and third decades when average values of 20 μm are not uncommon (Johnson et al., 1971) (Figure 54). It is at this age that the high serum calcium and phosphorus values of childhood fall and at the same time bone mass is maximal; the wide osteoid borders at this age may reflect a small lag between mineralization and new bone formation secondary to the comparatively

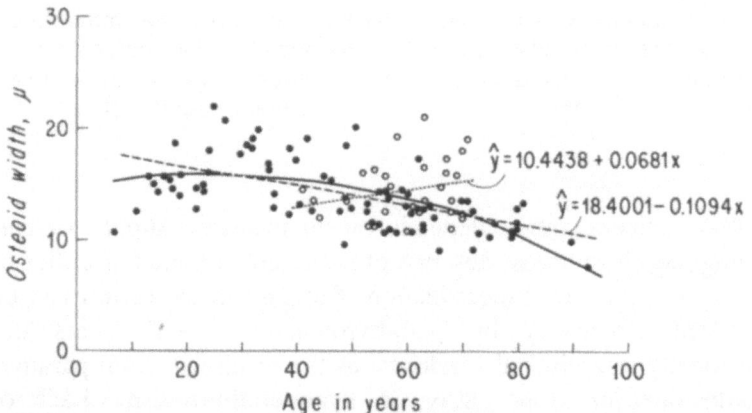

FIGURE 54. Variation in osteoid border thickness with age in normal individuals and in patients with osteoporosis. There is a tendency for osteoid width to decrease after the age of 20 in normal individuals. •=normal, o=osteoporotic, ———=normal regression line, ——— = normal best-fit curve, · · · · · =osteoporotic regression line.

large volume of new bone being formed. In the sixth and seventh decades, the width decreases again to values of approximately 10 to 12 μm. Individuals with osteoporosis, characterized by fractures of the spine or of the femoral neck, tend to have more osteoid tissue than a nonosteoporotic age-matched group (Johnson et al., 1971; Chalmers et al., 1969). Consequently, osteoporosis has been considered as a disorder of mineral metabolism, which is reflected in the wide osteoid borders. In the north of England there is no doubt that osteoporosis is frequently complicated by osteomalacia, since the amount of unmineralized osteoid is increased and the daily vitamin D intake is well below that recommended and probably below the amount which is ingested or to which the average person is exposed in the United States (Chalmers et al., 1969).

The cause of osteomalacia is a lack of the calcium and phosphorus needed for mineralization of the bone. A "dietary" deficiency of calcium is the most common cause of osteoporosis, and the deficiency is found to result in osteoporosis if it is mild and osteomalacia if excessive and accompanied by vitamin D lack. The dietary "deficiency" is generally evident only after metabolic or dietary abnormalities such as gastrectomy, sprue, or lactase deficiency, but in the case of osteoporosis, the nonpathological increases in osteoid tissue may be associated with mild calcium abnormalities such as a low milk intake or chronic vitamin D insufficiency. Unusual metabolic disturbances such as hypoparathyroidism, or hypophosphatemia, will also produce osteomalacia merely because there is insufficient calcium or phosphorus for the mineralization of the new tissue.

Renal failure in Europe is commonly associated with osteomalacia; there is a significant level of vitamin D insufficiency in the normal population in Europe which expresses itself as morphological osteomalacia when hyperphosphatemia further aggravates the insufficiency by retarding the 1,25-hydroxylation of vitamin D. Dialysis further exaggerates the osteomalacia either by further vitamin D depletion or by causing physiolog-

TABLE 15. Bone Changes in Normal, Uremic, and Dialyzed Uremic
Individuals[a]

Groups	Number	Hydroxyapatite (mg/ml bone)	Metacarpal cortical thickness (mm)	Osteoid thickness (μm^2)
Control individuals	15	255 ± 59	0.57 ± 0.08	8.0 ± 4.5
Uremic patients (no dialysis)	18	—	0.50 ± 0.05	12.1 ± 7.5
Uremic patients (dialysis)	65	148.7 ± 40.9	0.43 ± 0.10	17.3 ± 14.1

[a] From Ritz *et al.*, 1973.

ically significant hypophosphatemia (Table 15). The osteoid thickness is related to chemical determinations of bone density, although the latter would be a more insensitive measurement of the presence of unmineralized tissue.

SITE VARIATION AND TURNOVER CORRELATIONS

Site variation in dogs has been studied by a number of investigators. Marotti has determined the bone formation rates, with the help of tetracycline labeling, and has shown that these vary in different parts of the skeleton but that the variations are consistent (Marotti and DeLena, 1966a and b). Lee *et al.* (1965) showed the same consistency between different sites (Table 16). Nguyen and Jowsey (1970) have also shown a good correlation between bone formation in different areas of the skeleton, although surfaces rather than rates were determined in this study. Therefore, despite the large variation from site to site, a bone biopsy will reflect skeletal changes reliably, and values of bone turnover in two sites, provided they come from the same area, can be directly compared.

Bone formation values in a biopsy should correlate with other methods of evaluating bone formation. Unfortunately, there are none. The technique that approximates most closely the bone formation rates derived from surface measurements and the double tetracycline labeling determination of matrix deposition is the radiocalcium technique. If ^{45}Ca is injected intravenously into an animal the rate of disappearance of the isotope from the blood is a reflection of the urinary and fecal calcium excretion and the retention of calcium by bone. The calcium in bone is retained by deposition in mineral at sites of newborn formation and by long-term exchange. The former is obviously closely related to new bone deposition. A comparison of bone formation by the two methods shows that in bone with a high turnover rate the ^{45}Ca accretion rate and formation rate are similar (Table 17). However, in the adolescent dog in the cortical bone, the A-value is twice the bone formation value. and the adult would probably show a similar discrepency. The difference is not great, and the relationship between the two values lends credence to the bone formation data derived from biopsies (Shimmins et al., 1971).

The surface of bone that is covered by osteoid tissue is also a measure of osteomalacia. In normal bone this value is equal to the value for bone formation because osteoid is only present at

TABLE 16. Bone Formation Rates in Different Areas of the Skeleton in Two Different Dogs[a]

	Bone formation rate (%/day)	
	3-month-old puppy	9-month-old puppy
Femur, midshaft	1.7	0.07
Humerus, midshaft	1.3	0.08
Rib	3.4	0.56
Parietal bone	1.1	0.06
Iliac crest	—	1.45

[a] From Lee et al., 1965.

TABLE 17. Comparison of Accretion Rate, A,
Measured by ^{45}Ca Blood Disappearance and Bone
Formation Rate, F, Determined by Double
Tetracycline Labeling[a]

	A (%/day)	F (%/day)
3-month-old puppy		
Cortical bone	2.0	2.5
9-month-old puppy		
Cortical bone	0.30	0.16
Trabecular bone	0.77	0.82

[a] From Lee *et al.*, 1965.

sites of new bone formation. However, if there is a continued failure of mineralization then the unmineralized osteoid surface increases until in severe, chronic osteomalacia a large proportion of the bone becomes covered by osteoid. The measurement of the surface covered by osteoid varies from observer to observer because of the criteria used for recognizing the unmineralized matrix. The majority of investigators, for example, measure according to the presence of a translucent layer on the bone surface that contains lacunae and canaliculi (Johnson *et al.*, 1971; Chalmers *et al.*, 1967). However, in thin sections a very narrow layer of unmineralized matrix appears on virtually all bone surfaces (Raina, 1972). This layer is only 1 to 2 μm in thickness and probably does not represent any failure of normal mineralization, but it does have physiological significance as a differentiated layer that may separate bone from the extracellular fluid, and it provides a barrier between bone and the extracellular fluid.

Osteoid thickness of 10–15 μm are more usually encountered associated with bone formation. The surface covered by osteoid of this thickness or thicker represents new bone, either normally mineralized or, if the individual is osteomalacic, unmineralized. Increases above normal of the length of tissue covered by osteoid are the third and fourth steps of the development of osteomalacia and are generally greatly increased in symptomatic osteomalacia (Table 18). The surface multiplied by the thickness gives a value for osteoid volume, which is generally measured using a grid or point-count system. Measurements of the percentage of surface covered by inactive osteoid indicate the same defect in mineralization followed by the decrease in osteoblastic activity.

Correction of the factor causing osteomalacia will be seen first by the appearance of a mineralization front, then by a decrease in the width of unmineralized osteoid, and finally by decrease in the length of surface covered by osteoid. Healing of the bone lesion therefore occurs in reverse order of the appearance of the lesion.

Until recently osteocytes were considered to be inactive cells lying inertly within the mineralized matrix of bone. However, these cells have now been shown to be capable of resorptive activity that is termed osteocytic osteolysis, and less frequently they can be seen to lay down matrix, which becomes mineralized (Baud and Morgenthaler, 1963; Baud and Weber-Slatkine, 1961). Electron microscopic studies have clearly identified differences between the osteocytes in the various metabolic states; however, the majority of quantitative studies on

TABLE 18. Changes in Osteoid Surface and Volume in Two Patients[a]

	Before treatment	After treatment
Osteoid volume (%)		
Patient 1	48.2 ± 7.9	5.3 ± 0.6
Patient 2	84.4 ± 2.3	78.4 ± 4.1
Osteoid surface (%)		
Patient 1	89.6 ± 0.7	37.1 ± 5.5
Patient 2	95.1 ± 1.2	80.3 ± 10.4

[a] From Teitelbaum et al., 1976b. Values are mean ± SD.

bone biopsies have depended on measurements of the size of the osteocyte lacunae, which reflects parathyroid gland activity. By resorbing adjacent bone, the osteocytes are able to function like osteoclasts and because they lie within the mineralized matrix, they can be instrumental in returning calcium to the serum from the bone.

The average size of an osteocyte lacuna in adult human bone is $24 \times 15 \times 5$ μm. The size can be measured with an integrating eyepiece, or may more accurately be determined with an image-analyzing computer system (Meunier, 1973). Care must be taken with any osteocyte containing a nucleus if an automated method is used; any osteocyte lacuna not cut through its largest dimensions must be eliminated. A microradiograph of a 50 μm thick section would be the ideal preparation for measuring the size of osteocytes, since soft-tissue interference would be eliminated, and the majority of osteocytes are present in the bone section in their entirety (Jowsey et al., 1964). The manual method, which involves microscopic examination of the lacunae in 5 μm thick sections and measurement of the length and width of the lacunae, and the automatic method, using the Quantimet (automated scanning device), give similar and reliable data (Meunier and Bernard, 1976). The size in normal individuals is relatively constant in lamellar bone (Table 19) and does not vary with age or sex. Baud (1976) reported a decrease in both the number and size of osteocyte lacunae with age, however, the significance of the slope depends on only a few points and in the larger series of 92 reported by Meunier and Bernard (1976) there was no decrease with age, the size remaining constant. Baud suggested that the increased accuracy of the automated method may give the more accurate data.

Somewhat less satisfactory data have relied on separating osteocytes into "small," "large," and "empty" (Krempien et al., 1976). The separation is based on the characteristics of the lacuna and the presence or absence of a nucleus; the latter is clearly easy to define, however, the former depends to some extent on subjective evaluation. Nevertheless, the data derived in this way do not contradict direct quantitative measurements (Table 20).

TABLE 19. Osteocyte Size in Human Lamellar Bone [a]

	Number	Square micrometers (mean ± SD)
Control subjects	92	50.7 ± 5.5
Patients		
Primary hyperparathyroidism	91	64.2 ± 8.2
With adenomas	80	64.2 ± 8.2
With hyperplasia	9	65.3 ± 9.0

[a] From Meunier and Bernard, 1976.

TABLE 20. Percentage of Osteocytes That Are Small, Large, or Empty in Normal Bone and in Bone from Uremic Patients (Mean ± SD) [a]

	Control	Uremia
Haversian bone		
Small osteocytes	54.0 ± 8.3	31.2 ± 8.6[b]
Large osteocytes	39.2 ± 8.5	52.7 ± 8.7[b]
Empty osteocytes	60.1 ± 3.1	15.9 ± 9.0[b]
Interstitial bone		
Small osteocytes	35.6 ± 7.4	22.1 ± 9.2[b]
Large osteocytes	52.0 ± 6.1	56.3 ± 8.8[b]
Empty osteocytes	11.8 ± 5.1	21.1 ± 9.2[b]

[a] From Krempien, et al., 1976.
[b] Significantly different from control values.

Experimental studies in which dogs were fed a high phosphate diet to produce secondary hyperparathyroidism and in which osteocyte size increased indicated the role of the parathyroids in osteocytic osteolysis (Lok and Jaworski, 1976). Increases in osteocyte size in human bone is also associated with states of increased parathyroid activity, and it is probably true to say that osteocytic osteolysis reflects accurately elevated levels of serum parathyroid hormone.

A note of caution must be included: it is not possible to

prove that a large osteocyte was once smaller, and therefore it is not possible to *prove* that osteocytic osteolysis has occurred. By comparing normal and abnormal bone, a larger size can be fairly safely assumed to be a reflection of an increase in size, but it should be recognized that large osteocytes, which always were large, do occur in normal bone. They are found in woven bone as seen in Figure 9b and can clearly be distinguished from osteocytic osteolysis since they are predictably found between osteones in woven bone of a high mineral and glycosamin-oglycan content. In normal bone the number of large osteocytes are more frequent in Haversian bone than in interstitial bone (Table 20).

Volume changes in bone have already been referred to in the discussion of trabecular and cortical bone. Measurements of trabecular bone volume, determined with a point-count method, have uniformly demonstrated a decrease with age in human beings (Table 21). Meunier has used a point-count method by which the percentage of intersections falling on bone are an estimate of bone area. If the section is infinitely thin, the measurement can be extrapolated to volume (Meunier and Courpron, 1976). There is a good correlation between trabecular bone volume, obtained in this way, in different sites (Table 22). An automated method may also be used. The first reports were derived from the use of a computerized scanning camera that analyzes 500,000 picture points (Meunier, 1973). In a mineralized section stained purple with solochrome-cyanin, the image analyzer (Quantimet-720) can differentiate fairly well between bone and soft tissue. The major error probably arises from the imperfection of the section which may have rents and fractures or dark-staining soft tissue (Figure 44). The method is more rapid than the manual method, but subject to more error. A microradiograph provides a better image for a computerized scanning image analyzing system, since the bone is white and the "nonbone" black. In this method referred to as videodensitometry, 1,000,000 8-bit picture elements are analyzed from a photographic enlargement of the microradiograph (Figure 55).

TABLE 21. Trabecular Bone Volume Changes with Age (Percent, mean ± SD)

Study	Age in Years							
	15–19	20–29	30–39	40–49	50–59	60–69	70–79	80–89
Meunier & Courpron (1976)	23.2 ± 2.8	22.9 ± 5.2	21.4 ± 4.5	20.4 ± 2.8	19.4 ± 3.4	15.1 ± 3.1	16.9 ± 3.7	15.3 ± 3.0
Schulz & Delling (1976a)	20.7 ± 3.1	20.4 ± 4.0	20.0 ± 3.2	19.9 ± 4.6	18.6 ± 5.2	15.2 ± 4.8	14.2 ± 5.5	11.1 ± 3.0
Jowsey (1977b) Trabecular bone	25.5 ± 3.3	23.4 ± 7.9	20.8 ± 4.2	16.3 ± 4.7	17.5 ± 5.2	13.0 ± 4.6	14.2 ± 5.2	12.4 ± 4.2
Jowsey (1977b) Cortical bone	84.6 ± 5.2	87.6 ± 3.4	83.5 ± 5.4	64.3 ± 8.9	65.7 ± 8.9	52.7 ± 14.0	54.5 ± 23.0	44.9 ± 15.2

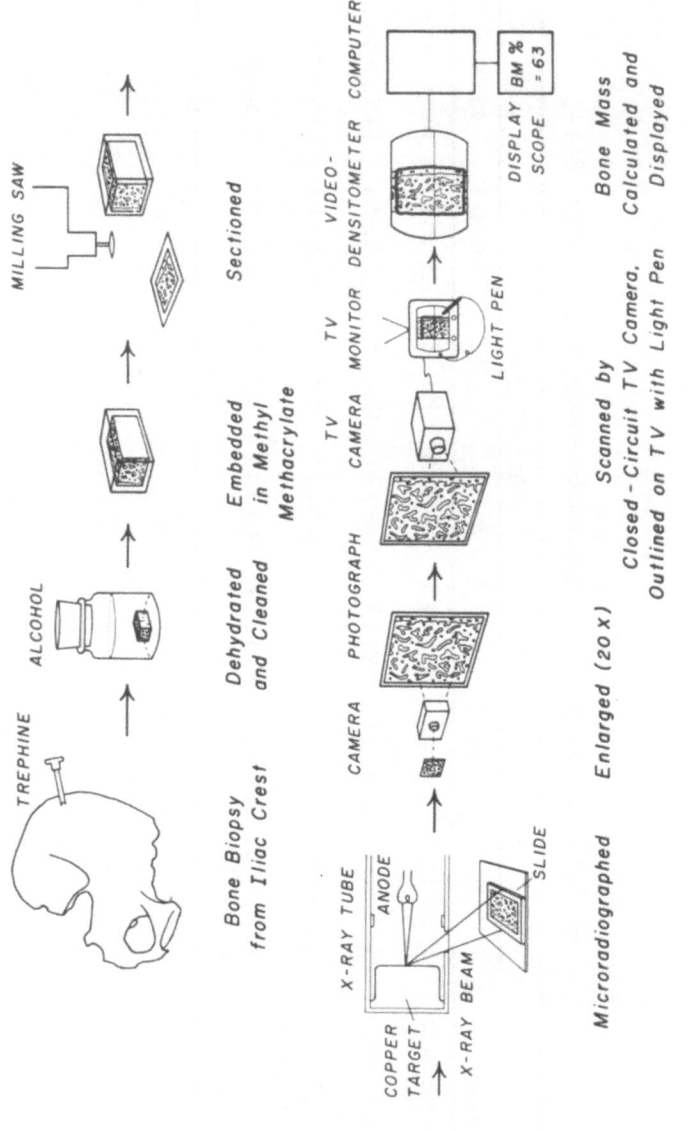

FIGURE 55. Method for measurement of bone mass by digital scanning videodensitometry. Diagram to show the procedure for making videodensitometric measurements of bone density in microradiographs of sections of the iliac crest.

TABLE 22. Trabecular Bone Volume Measurements in Different
Sites[a]

	n	r	p
Transverse iliac crest (Fig. 26b)			
vs. vertical iliac crest (Fig. 26a)	86	0.63	<.001
Transverse iliac crest (Fig. 26b)			
vs. lumbar vertebra	45	0.78	<.001

[a] From Meunier and Courpron, 1976.

TABLE 23. Repeatability of Videodensitometry Technique in
32 Sections of an Iliac Crest Biopsy

	Percentage of bone in section (type Fig. 26d)		
	Mean	SD	SE
10-year-old control male	24.4	1.6	0.27
6-year-old control male	40.8	2.1	0.37

This permits both greater resolution and a complete separation
of mineralized and nonmineralized structures since the print,
which is the image scanned, can be photographically made
black and white, rather than different shades of gray (Robb *et
al.*, 1973). The reproducibility of the data is excellent, and
meaningful changes in bone mass can be obtained (Table 23)
(Figure 56). Increase in trabecular and cortical bone volume
have been demonstrated in patients with multiple myeloma and
in patients with osteoporosis treated with fluoride and calcium
(Kyle *et al.*, 1975).

A similar technique has been used by Garrick and co-
workers (Garrick *et al.*, 1972) using an iliac crest biopsy of the

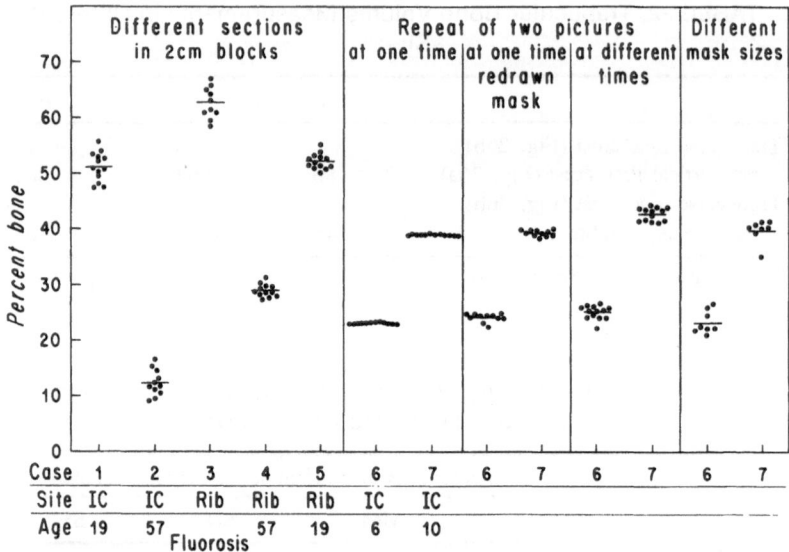

FIGURE 56. Variance in the videodensitometric analysis of bone density.

superior spine (Figure 26a). The repeatability is good, the observer and technique error being small and the reproducibility between different specimens of the same iliac crest and between the iliac crests on the left and right side giving standard deviations of 2.2 or less with bone mass measurements of about 20 to 30%.

Chapter 7

Bone Biopsy Results in Pathological Conditions

It would be beyond the scope of this book to describe the changes in osteoid, bone formation and resorption, bone volume, and the other parameters measured in bone biopsies. However, it is appropriate to describe some results of biopsy procedures to illustrate the problems that arise in analyses of bone biopsies and in understanding the data reported in the literature.

A comparison of the results described by different investigators vary for a number of different reasons. Patients with osteoporosis frequently seek medical aid as a result of a fracture and may be hospitalized and studied under hospital conditions. Both the fracture and resulting pain and the hospital stay will cause a decrease in bone formation which is visible after 4–18 h of bed rest (Jowsey, 1977a). As a result, both osteoporotic individuals and individuals who have been at bed rest, or normal people who are staying in a hospital for observation, will show a depressed bone formation value (Table 24).

A second cause of apparent controversy is the difference between the site of the biopsy analyzed. Essentially all biopsies are from the iliac crest; some investigators analyze only trabecular bone. This results in a difference in bone formation values

TABLE 24. Variation in Bone Formation and Resorption in Cortical and Trabecular Bone, Evaluated by Quantitative Microradiography in Normal and Osteoporotic Individuals, under Normal Activity and Conditions and after 1 to 17 Days of Bedrest

	Number	Percentage formation	Number	Percentage resorption
Normals				
Bed rest	21	0.7 ± 0.5^a	18	4.1 ± 2.3
Normal activity	21	2.4 ± 0.4	18	5.6 ± 1.2
Osteoporotics				
Bed rest	6	0.3 ± 0.2	6	16.4 ± 5.6
Normal activity	27	2.1 ± 1.3	27	8.4 ± 4.4

^{a} Values are mean $\pm$ SD.

which tend to decrease in trabecular bone with age but remain constant if both cortical and trabecular bone are analyzed (Figure 24). Bone resorption in trabecular bone has been reported to remain constant with age or to increase with age after skeletal maturity is reached. Constant and increasing age-related values are both reported in trabecular bone in the iliac crest, while increasing values are reported in trabecular and cortical bone of the iliac crest (Table 25). The differences appear mainly to be the result of the greater response of the cortical bone to a metabolic abnormality. Teitelbaum also observed this in cortical bone of osteoporotic patients, those with higher serum parathyroid levels showing greater cortical bone resorption values while trabecular bone resorption did not increase (Teitelbaum et al., 1976a). Bone resorption values measured in trabecular bone by other investigators does not show an increase in osteoporotic individuals. In a group of young patients with osteoporosis (age range 19–45), Bordier found resorption to be increased, although the variation in the control and patient groups was large enough to prevent any statistical difference (Bordier et al., 1973b) (Table 26). Older individuals with osteoporosis also showed an increase in resorption compared with an age-matched normal group (Bordier et al., 1964). However, the latter data

TABLE 25. Bone Resorption Values in Trabecular or Trabecular and Cortical Iliac Crest (IC) and Cortical Rib (R) Specimens in Different Aged Normal Individuals (Mean ± SD)

Study	Age:	Bone resorption values					
		30–39	40–49	50–59	60–69	70–79	80–89
Schenk et al. (1969)							
IC trabecular bone[a]		2.7 ± 1.8	2.6 ± 3.1	2.5 ± 2.1	2.7 ± 2.5	2.7 ± 2.1	—
Schulz & Delling (1976c)							
IC trabecular bone[a]		6.4 ± 2.7	5.3 ± 4.1	9.4 ± 5.5	7.5 ± 5.2	9.3 ± 7.5	9.8 ± 4.0
Jowsey (1977b)							
IC trabecular and cortical bone[c]		3.0 ± 0.8	3.8 ± 0.9	3.8 ± 1.9	3.9 ± 1.3	4.5 ± 1.7	3.7 ± 0.9
Sedlin et al. (1963)							
R cortical bone[b]		0.28 ± 0.21	0.27 ± 0.18	0.46 ± 0.30	0.60 ± 0.30	0.40 ± 0.21	—
Meunier et al. (1973a)							
IC trabecular bone[c]		4.1 ± 0.8	3.9 ± 1.1	3.6 ± 1.2	3.9 ± 1.1	3.9 ± 0.9	—

[a] Osteoclast index (number of osteoclasts divided by surface density).
[b] Values are spaces/mm ^{2}, mean ± SE.
[c] Percentage of surface undergoing resorption.

TABLE 26. Bone Resorption in Iliac Crest Biopsies
of Control and Osteoporotic Individuals (Mean ± SD)

Study	Control	Osteoporosis
Schenk et al. (1972)[a]	0.6 ± 0.46	0.5 ± 0.41
Bordier et al. (1973b)[a]	0.59 ± 0.52	0.95 ± 0.86
Meunier et al. (1973a)[b]	3.64 ± 1.12	3.30 ± 1.24
Jowsey (1977b)[c]	3.9 ± 1.40	10.3 ± 5.43

[a] Percentage of trabecular surface covered with osteoclasts.
[b] Percentage of trabecular surface with Howship's lacunae (resorption osteo-clastic trabecular surface).
[c] Percentage of cortical and trabecular surface with osteoclasts.

were derived from measuring Howship's lacunae and not os-teoclasts. Nevertheless, the authors conclude that resorption is increased in osteoporosis and is responsible for the bone loss in this disease. Later data from the same authors indicate that resorption is not increased in osteoporosis (Bordier and Tun Chot, 1972); the later data were presumably derived from os-teoclast counts, which explained the change in the opinion of these authors of the pathogenesis of this disease.

In some studies, apparently comparable groups do show significant difference because of previous treatment of the pa-tients, which the investigators think not to have an effect on bone metabolism. In a group of osteoporotic patients reported by Jett and co-workers (Jett et al., 1967) one-third of the pa-tients had received calcium treatment, which is known to cause a decrease in bone formation (Riggs et al., 1976). Jett reported that bone formation was low normal in osteoporosis, a finding consistent with other studies but no doubt dependent to some extent on the previous treatment received by some (30%) of the patients. Other investigators fail to distinguish between different metabolic conditions; for example, patients with chronic renal failure and uremia are a totally different group of individuals from patients with chronic renal failure who are on dialysis.

Variations in populations may also occur as a result of the

rigorousness with which the patients are selected. For example, of the 18 patients with osteoporosis reported by Jett *et al.* (1967) only 3 patients had no associated medical problems, all others having had either treatment of some kind or hip fractures, multiple fractures, or gastrectomy which would inevitably result in alterations in bone metabolism. The same is true of control groups. Rigorous selection of normal individuals frequently results in a change in the mean and range of the control data (Table 27). Even the occupation of the control or patient group may alter the data; for example, in a control group of males with active employment with an average age of 60 years, the bone density measured by videodensitometry was 81%, while a group of mainly sedentary workers demonstrated a bone density of 61%.

Probably the most useful information to be derived from bone biopsy studies has been the data derived by a single group of investigators using one method and comparing patients with controls or patients before and after treatment. All variations resulting from technique are eliminated. Perhaps most work has been carried out on patients with different disorders of bone, the bone biopsies being taken to determine whether bone loss is the result of increased resorption as in osteoporosis (Table 28) or

TABLE 27. Bone Resorption and Formation in
Control Populations

Year	Bone resorption	Bone formation
1965[a]	8.5 ± 3.1[c]	2.6 ± 1.2
1976[b]	3.9 ± 1.4	2.0 ± 1.4

[a] 1965 controls were an unselected group; corpses brought into the morgues of three major U.S. cities.
[b] 1976 controls were a highly selected group of deaths by accident or acute CVA with proven physical activity at the time of death and an extensive pathology report allowing exclusion of liver disease, parathyroid gland size increase, etc.
[c] Values are mean ± SD, percentage of total surface.

TABLE 28. Bone Resorption in Control and
Osteoporotic Individuals Measured by
Quantitative Microradiography

Age, years	Control	Osteoporotic
30–39	3.0 ± 0.8^a	9.4 ± 3.1
40–49	3.8 ± 0.9	9.4 ± 4.4
50–59	3.8 ± 1.9	9.9 ± 5.4
60–69	3.9 ± 1.3	10.5 ± 5.2
70–79	4.5 ± 1.7	11.9 ± 5.0
80–89	3.7 ± 0.9	16.6 ± 8.5

[a] Values are resorption percentage of total surface, mean ±
SD.

TABLE 29. Bone Turnover in Metabolic Bone Disease and Normals
(Mean ± SD)

	Number	Bone formation (%)	Bone resorption (%)
Disease			
Hypoparathyroidism (IC)	5	0.7 ± 0.4	0.5 ± 1.0
Hyperparathyroidism (PIC)[a]	24	3.7 ± 3.3	13.0 ± 4.3
Paget's (IC)	13	12.6 ± 9.5	22.8 ± 11.0
Hypercortisonism (IC)	26	0.2 ± 0.2	11.4 ± 4.6
Osteoporosis (IC)	168	2.7 ± 1.9	10.8 ± 5.3
Normals (IC)	153	3.2 ± 2.7	4.9 ± 2.6

[a] Posterior iliac crest.

decreased formation and increased resorption, as in hypercor-
tisonism (Table 29). In single-patient groups the effect of therapy can also be evaluated by comparing biopsies before and
after treatment, and the metabolic change in bone can be evaluated long before any change in the radiological appearance is
seen (Table 30).

TABLE 30. The Effect of Various Therapeutic Agents on Bone Formation and Resorption in Osteoporotic Individuals

	Pretreatment		After 3–4 months		After 1–2 years	
	Formation	Resorption	Formation	Resorption	Formation	Resorption
EHDP	1.7	10.0	0.7	10.0	1.0	7.2
Estrogens	4.8	15.0	4.0	6.4^a	0.7^b	10.4^b
Anabolic agents	2.5	11.1	3.2	9.5	0.8^b	8.7
Calcitonin	2.2	11.6	1.7	14.9		
Calcium infusions	2.1	9.5	3.9	5.5^a		
Oral phosphate	3.8	11.0	2.3	17.4^a	0.7^b	16.8^b
Fluoride and calcium (osteoporosis)	2.6	13.5	9.4^a	11.5^a	4.4^b	4.7^b
Fluoride and calcium (myeloma)	3.6				8.1^a	

[a] Significantly different from pretreatment value.
[b] Significantly different from short-term therapy value.

Chapter 8

Conclusions

The major problems in bone biopsy procedures have been the variation in the type of bone analyzed and the parameters in which the results are expressed. The former results in different data for legitimate reasons because trabecular and cortical bone behave differently and lead to different quantitative results. The latter leads to confusion among those not familiar with morphometric techniques and requires a perhaps unreasonable effort in understanding the differences between different sets of data.

Nevertheless, the advantage of quantitative morphometric methods is self-evident. A biopsy report as follows is not overly helpful:

> The specimen consists of three irregular, somewhat cylindrical portions of cancellous appearing bone. They are submitted intact for decalcification prior to sectioning. The sections indicate cancellous bone with no diagnostic alterations and the bony spicules are histologically unremarkable.

In contrast, a quantitative evaluation of undemineralized bone from the same patient might read:

Parameter	Value	Normal age-matched group
Bone formation, %	2.3	2.1 ± 1.0
Bone resorption, %	11.7	4.2 ± 1.8
Osteoid surface. %	17	2.1 ± 1.0
Osteoid border width, μm	27.2	15.0 ± 2.3
Mineralization front, %	40	83 ± 10.2

This would indicate no abnormality of formation, a raised resorption level, and a defect in mineralization and it would lead the physician to investigate vitamin D metabolism in the patient and to measure a serum parathyroid hormone level.

Quantitative morphometric analyses of bone biopsies are more frequently carried out, and partly because the data have proved useful, bone biopsies are being taken more frequently in patients with metabolic bone disease.

References

Ball, J. (1957) A simple method of defining osteoid in undecalcified sections. *J. Clin. Pathol.* **10:**281–282.

Barer, M., and Jowsey, J. (1967) Bone formation and resorption in osteoporosis. *Clin. Orthop.* **52:**241–247.

Baud, C. A. (1976) Histophysiology of the osteocyte: An introduction to the morphometry of peri-osteocytic lacunae. In *Bone Morphometry.* Edited by Z. F. G. Jaworski. Univ. of Ottawa Press, Ottawa, pp. 267–272.

Baud, C. A., and Auil, E. (1971) Ostocyte differential count in normal human alveolar bone. *Acta Anat.* **78:**321–327.

Baud, C. A., and Dupont, D. H. (1962) The fine structure of the osteocytes in the adult compact bone. *5th Int. Congress Electron Microscopy,* p. 10.

Baud, C. A., and Morgenthaler, P. W. (1963) The submicroscopic channels in bone tissue. *XVI Int. Congress Zool. Proc.* **2:**313.

Baud, C. A., and Weber-Slatkine, S. (1961) Aspects microscopiques et submicroscopiques des ostéoplastes du tissu osseux compact. *Bull. Micr. Appl.* **11:**73–76.

Bohatirchuk, F. (1966) Calciolysis as the initial stage of bone resorption. *Amer. J. Med.* **41:**836–846.

Bonucci, E. (1974) The organic–inorganic relationships in bone matrix undergoing osteoclastic resorption. *Calcif. Tiss. Res.* **16:**13–36.

Bordier, Ph. J., and Tun Chot, S. (1972) Quantitative histology of metabolic bone disease. *Clin. Endocrinol. Metab.* **1:**197–215.

Bordier, Ph., J. and Tun Chot, S. (1973) Histological aspects of bone remodelling, with special reference to the effects of parathyroid hormone and vitamin D. *Excerpta Medica Int. Congress Series 270,* pp. 95–102.

Bordier, Ph. J., Matrajt, H., Miravet, L., and Hioco, D. (1964) Mésure histologique de la masse et de la résorption des travées osseuses. *Pathol. Biol.* **12**:1238–1243.

Bordier, Ph. J., Tun Chot, S., and Marie, P. (1972) Unpublished data.

Bordier, Ph. J., Arnaud, C., Hawker, C., Tun Chot, S. and Hioco, D. (1973a) Relationship between serum immunoreactive parathyroid hormone, osteoclastic and osteocytic bone resorptions and serum calcium in primary hyperparathyroidism and osteomalacia. *Excerpta Medica International Congress Series 270*: 222–228.

Bordier, Ph. J., Miravet, L., Hioco, D. (1973b) Young adult osteoporosis. *Clin. Endocrinol. Metab.* **2**:277–292.

Buring, K. (1975) On the origin of cells in heterotopic bone formation. *Clin. Orthop.* **110**:293–302.

Burkhart, J. M., and Jowsey, J. (1966) Morphologic evidence of osteomalacia in the parathyroidectomized dog. *Mayo Clin. Proc.* **41**:663–667.

Byers, P. D., and Smith, R. (1967) New appliance—Trephine for full-thickness iliac-crest biopsy. *Brit. Med. J.* **1**:682–683.

Cabanela, M. E., and Jowsey, J. (1974) Effect of ethane-1-hydroxy-1, diphosphonate on bone turnover in adult dogs. *Clin. Orthop.* **100**:364–369.

Chalmers, J., Conacher, W. D., Gardner, D. L., and Scott, P. J. (1967) Osteoporosis—a common disease in elderly women. *J. Bone Joint Surg.* **49B**:403–423.

Chalmers, J., Barclay, A., Davidson, A. M., Macleod, D. A. D., and Williams, D. A. (1969) Quantitative measurements of osteoid in health and disease. *Clin. Orthop.* **63**:196–209.

Ch'uan, C. H. (1931) Mitochondria in osteoclasts. *Anat. Rec.* **49**:397–401.

Connor, T. B., Freijanes, J., Stoner, R. E., Martin, L. G., and Jowsey, J. (1974) Generalized osteosclerosis in primary hyperparathyroidism. *Trans. Amer. Clin. Climatol. Assoc.* **85**:185–201.

Courpron, P., Giroud, J. M., Bringuier, J. P., and Meunier, P. (1974) Histomorphometry of iliac spongy bone. The influence of preparation and quantitative analysis techniques on the measurement of iliac trabecular bone volume. *Lyon Med.* **232**:515–522.

Debnam, J. W., and Staple, T. W. (1975a) Needle biopsy of bone. *Radiol. Clin. North Amer.* **13**:157–164.

Debnam, J. W., and Staple, T. W. (1975b) Trephine bone biopsy by radiologists. *Radiology* **116**:607–609.

Dekker, G., Eggink, C. O., and Verhaar, T. H. C. (1968) An instrument for obtaining bone specimens for patho-histologic examination. Excerpta Medica, *Medical Instrumentation* sectie **27**:2.

Duursma, S. A., Visser, W. J., Zoeren, M. V., and Korver, F. (1969) A bone biopsy procedure. *Calcif. Tiss. Res.* **4**:269–273.

Evarts, C. Mc. (1975) Diagnostic techniques: Closed biopsy of bone. *Clin. Orthop.* **107**:100–111.

Fornasier, V. L., and Vilaghy, M. I. (1973) Laboratory suggestions: The results of bone biopsy with a new instrument. *Amer. J. Clin. Pathol.* **60:**570–573.

Frost, H. M. (1958) Preparation of thin undecalcified sections by rapid manual method. *Stain Technol.* **33:** 273–277.

Frost, H. M. (1959) Staining of fresh, undecalcified, thin bone sections. *Stain Technol.* **34:**135–146.

Frost, H. M. (1960) Lamellar osteoid mineralized per day in man. *Henry Ford Hosp. Med. Bull.* **8:**267–272.

Frost, H. M., and Villanueva, A. R. (1961) Human osteoblastic activity—Part I. A comparative method of measurement with some results. *Henry Ford Hosp. Med. Bull.* **9:**76–86.

Garrick, R., Doman, P., and Posen, S. (1972) Quantitative histology of bone: The use of a computer program and results in normal subjects. *Clin. Sci.* **43:**789–797.

Gothlin, G., and Ericsson, J. L. E. (1973) On the histogenesis of the cells in fracture callus. *Virchows Arch. Abt. B. Zellpath.* **12:**318–329.

Howell, D. S. (1976) Calcification mechanisms. *Isr. J. Med. Sci.* **12:**91–97.

Jande, S. S. (1971) Fine structural study of osteocytes and their surrounding bone matrix with respect to their age in young chicks. *J. Ultrastruct. Res.* **37:**279–300.

Jande, S. S., and Bélanger, L. F. (1973) The life cycle of the osteocyte. *Clin. Orthop.* **94:**281–305.

Jaworski, Z. F., and Lok, E. (1972) The rate of osteoclastic bone erosion in Haversian remodeling sites of adult dog's rib. *Calcif. Tiss. Res.* **10:**103–112.

Jaworski, Z. F. G., and Lok, E. (1976) The effect of moderate uremia and high phosphate-normal calcium diet on the linear erosion rate measured in the Haversian turnover sites in the rib of the adult dog. In *Bone Morphometry*. Edited by Z. F. G. Jaworski. Univ. of Ottawa Press, Ottawa, pp. 148–152.

Jaworski, Z. F. G., Lok, E., and Wellington, J. L. (1975) Impaired osteoclastic function and linear bond erosion rate in secondary hyperparathyroidism associated with chronic renal failure. *Clin. Orthop.* **107:**289–310.

Jett, S., Wu, K., and Frost, H. M. (1967) Tetracycline-based histological measurement of cortical–endosteal bone formation in normal and osteoporotic rib. *Henry Ford Hosp. Med. J.* **15:**325–344.

Johnson, K. A., Riggs, B. L., Kelly, P. J., and Jowsey, J. (1971) Osteoid tissue in normal and osteoporotic individuals. *J. Clin. Endocrinol. Metab.* **33:**745–751.

Johnson, K. A., Kelly, P. J., and Jowsey, J. (1977) Percutaneous biopsy of the iliac crest. *Clin. Orthop. Relat. Res.* **123:**34–36.

Johnson, L. C. (1964) Morphologic analysis in pathology. In *Bone Biodynamics*. Edited by H. F. Frost. Little, Brown, Boston, pp. 543–654.

Jowsey, J. (1966) Studies of Haversian systems in man and some animals. *J. Anat.* **100:**857–864.

Jowsey, J. (1973a) Autoradiographic and microradiographic studies of bone. In *Biological Mineralization*. Edited by I. Zipkin. John Wiley & Sons, New York, pp. 297–333.

Jowsey, J. (1973b) Microradiography: A morphologic approach to quantitating bone turnover. *Excerpta Medica, International Congress Series* **270:**114–123.

Jowsey, J. (1977a) *Metabolic Diseases of Bone.* W. B. Saunders, Philadelphia.

Jowsey, J. (1977b) Unpublished data.

Jowsey, J., Riggs, B. L., and Kelly, P. J. (1964) Mineral metabolism in osteocytes. *Mayo Clin. Proc.* **39:**480–484.

Jowsey, J., Kelly, P. J., Riggs, B. L., Bianco, A. J., Scholz, D. A., and Gershon-Cohen, J. (1965) Quantitative microradiographic studies of normal and osteoporotic bone. *J. Bone Joint Surg.* **47A:**785–806.

Jowsey, J., Holley, K. E., and Linman, J. W. (1970) Effect of sodium etidronate in adult cats. *J. Lab. Clin. Med.* **76:**126–133.

Jowsey, J., Riggs, B. L., Kelly, P. J., Hoffman, D. L., and Bordier, Ph. (1971) The treatment of osteoporosis with disodium ethane-1-hydroxy-1, 1-diphosphonate. *J. Lab. Clin. Med.* **78:**574–584.

Kahn, A. J., and Simmons, D. J. (1975) Investigation of cell lineage in bone using a chimaera of chick and quail embryonic tissue. *Nature (London)* **258:**325–327.

Kelly, P. J., Jowsey, J., and Riggs, B. L. (1965) A comparison of different metabolic methods of determining bone formation. *Clin. Orthop.* **40:**7–11.

Krempien, B., Ritz, E., and Geiger, G. (1976) Behaviour of osteocytes in various ages and chronic uremia. Morphological studies in human cortical bone. In *Bone Morphometry*. Edited by Z. F. G. Jaworski. Univ. of Ottawa Press, Ottawa. pp. 288–296.

Kyle, R. A., Jowsey, J., Kelly, P. J., and Taves, D. R. (1975) Multiple-myeloma bone disease: The comparative effect of sodium fluoride and calcium carbonate or placebo. *N. Engl. J. Med.* **293:**1334–1338.

Landeros, O., and Frost, H. M. (1964) The cross section size of the osteon. *Henry Ford Hosp. Bull.* **12:**517–525.

Lee, W. R., Marshall, J. H., and Sissons, H. A. (1965) Calcium accretion and bone formation in dogs. *J. Bone Joint Surg.* **47B:**157–180.

Little, D. A. (1972) Bone biopsy on cattle and sheep for studies of phosphorus status. *Aust. Vet. J.* **48:**668–670.

Lok, E., and Jaworski, Z.F.G. (1976) Changes in the periosteocytic lacunae size observed under the experimental conditions in the adult dog. In *Bone Morphometry*. Edited by Z.F.G. Jaworski. Univ. of Ottawa Press, Ottawa, pp. 297–300.

Lucht, U. (1972) Absorption of peroxidase by osteoclasts as studied by electron microscope histochemistry. *Histochemie* **29**:274–286.

Marotti, G., and DeLena, M. (1966a) Analisi quantitativa dei processi di ricostruzione strutturale nella mandibola del cane in rapporto all'eta. *Anat. Embriol.* **71**:229.

Marotti, G., and DeLena, M. (1966b) Il rinnovamento della spurnosa delle vertebre in cani di varia eta. *La Clin. Ortoped.* **18**:518.

Merz, W. A., and Schenk, R. K. (1970) A quantitative histological study on bone formation in human cancellous bone. *Acta Anat.* **76**:1–15.

Meunier, P. (1973) Use of an image analyzing computer for bone morphometry. *Excerpta Medica Int. Congress Series 270*, pp. 148–151.

Meunier, P. and Edouard, C. (1973). Personal communication.

Meunier, P., and Bernard, J. (1976) Morphometric analysis of periosteocytic osteolysis. In *Bone Morphometry*. Edited by Z. F. G. Jaworski. Univ. of Ottawa Press, Ottawa, pp. 279–287.

Meunier, P., and Courpron, P. (1976) Iliac trabecular bone volume in 236 controls—representativeness of iliac samples. In *Bone Morphometry*. Edited by Z. F. G. Jaworski. Univ. of Ottawa Press, Ottawa, pp. 100–105.

Meunier, P., Courpron, P., Edouard, C., Bernard, J., Bringuier, J., and Vignon, G. (1973a) Physiological senile involution and pathological rarefaction of bone. *Clin. Endocrinol. Metab.* **2**:239–256.

Meunier, P., Vignon, G., Bernard, J., Edouard, C., and Courpron, P. (1973b) Quantitative bone histology as applied to the diagnosis of hyperparathyroid states. *Excerpta Medica Int. Congress Series 270*, pp. 215–221.

Meyer, P. C. (1956) The histological identification of osteoid tissue. *J. Pathol. Bacteriol.* **71**:325–333.

Mundy, G. R., Raisz, L. G., Cooper, R. A., Schechter, G. P., and Salmon, S. E. (1974) Evidence for the secretion of an osteoclast stimulating factor in myeloma. *N. Engl. J. Med.* **291**:1041–1046.

Nguyen, V., and Jowsey, J. (1970) A study of bone formation in dogs of different metabolic states using autoradiographic visualization of ^{45}Ca. *Acta Orthop. Scand.* **40**:708–720.

Owen, M. (1971) Cellular dynamics of bone. In *The Biochemistry and Physiology of Bone*, Vol. III. Edited by G. H. Bourne, 2nd Ed.. Academic Press, New York/London, pp. 271–298.

Owen, M., and Shetlar, M. R. (1968) Uptake of ^3H-glucosamine by osteoclasts. *Nature (London)* **220**:*1335*–1336.

Parfitt, A. M. (1973) The quantitative approach to bone morphology. A critique of current methods and their interpretation. *Excerpta Medica Int. Congress Series 270*, pp. 86–94.

Pawlicki, R. (1975) Bone canaliculus endings in the area of the osteocyte lacuna. *Acta Anat.* **91**:292–303.

Raina, V. (1972) Normal osteoid tissue. *J. Clin. Pathol.* **25**:229–232.

Raina, V. (1973) Rickets and osteomalacia—a morphological study. *Indian J. Med. Res.* **61**:190–194.

Rasmussen, H., and Bordier, Ph. (1973) The cellular basis of metabolic bone disease. *N. Engl. J. Med.* **289**:25–32.

Recklinhausen, F. von (1910) *Rachitis und osteomalacia.* Gustav Fisher, Jena.

Remagen, W., Hohling, J. J., Hall, T. A., and Caesar, R. (1969) Electron microscopical and microprobe observations on the cell sheath of stimulated osteocytes. *Calcif. Tiss. Res.* **4**:60–68.

Riggs, B. L., Kelly, P. J., Jowsey, J. and Keating, F. R. (1965) Skeletal alterations in hyperparathyroidism, determinations of bone formation, resorption, and morphologic changes by microradiography. *J. Clin. Endocrinol.* **25**:777–783.

Riggs, B. L., Jowsey, J., Kelly, P. J., Hoffman, D. L., and Arnaud, C. D. (1976) Effects of oral therapy with calcium and vitamin D in primary osteoporosis. *J. Clin. Endocrinol. Metab.* **42**:1139–1144.

Ritz, E., Krempien, B., Mehls, O., and Bommer, J. (1973) Dialysis bone disease. *Excerpta Medica Int. Congress Series 270*:616–620.

Robb, R. A., Johnson, S. A., Greenleaf, J. F., Wondrow, M. A., and Wood, E. H. (1973) An operator-interactive computer-controlled system for high-fidelity digitization and analysis of biomedical images. *Photo-Optical Instumentation Engineers Seminar on Quantitative Imagery in the Biomedical Sciences-II,* **40**:11–26.

Sacker, L. S., and Nordin, B. E. C. (1954) A simple bone biopsy needle. *Nature (London)* **1**:347.

Salassa, R. M., Jowsey, J., and Arnaud, C. D. (1970) Hypophosphatemic osteomalacia associated with "nonendocrine" tumors. *N. Engl. J. Med.* **283**:65–70.

Schenk, R. K., Merz, W. A., and Müller, J. (1969) A quantitative histological study on bone resorption in human cancellous bone. *Acta. Anat.* **74**:44–53.

Schenk, R. K., Olah, A. J., and Merz, W. A. (1973) Bone cell counts. *Excerpta Medica Int. Congress Series 270*:103–113.

Schenk, R. K. (1976) Standard values—(histomorphometry) iliac crest cancellous bone. In *Bone Morphometry.* Edited by Z. F. G. Jaworski. Univ. of Ottawa Press, Ottawa, pp. 392–394.

Schulz, A., and Delling, G. (1976a) Histomorphometric preparation and technique determination of trabecular bone volume. In *Bone Morphometry.*

Edited by Z. F. G. Jaworski. Univ. of Ottawa Press, Ottawa, pp. 106–108.

Schulz, A., and Delling, G. (1976b) Age-related changes of new bone formation—determination of histomorphometric parameters of the iliac crest trabecular bone. In *Bone Morphometry*. Edited by Z. F. G. Jaworski. Univ. of Ottawa Press, Ottawa, pp. 189–190.

Schulz, A., and Delling, G. (1976c) Age-related changes of bone resorption parameters in iliac crest trabecular bone. In *Bone Morphometry*. Edited by Z. F. G. Jaworski. Univ. of Ottawa Press, Ottawa, pp. 161–162.

Sedlin, E. D., Frost, H. M., and Villanueva, A. R. (1963) Age changes in resorption in human rib cortex. *J. Gerontol.* **18:**345–349.

Sherrard, D., Baylink, D., and Wergedal, J. (1972) Bone disease in uremia. *Trans. Amer. Soc. Artif. Intern. Organs* **28:**412–415.

Sherrard, D. J., Baylink, D. J., Wergedal, J., and Maloney, N. (1973) Increased bone formation rate in uremia. *Excerpta Medica Int. Congress Series 270*, pp. 612–615.

Sherrard, D. J., Baylink, D. J., Wergedal, J. E., and Maloney, N. A. (1974) Quantitative histological studies on the pathogenesis of uremic bone disease. *J. Clin. Endocrinol. Metab.* **39:**119–135.

Shimmins, J., Lee, W. R., Smith, D. A., and Lucie, N. (1971) A study of calcium deposition in the skeleton of a dog using autoradiography. *Calcif. Tiss. Res.* **8:**121–132.

Singh, M., Riggs, B. L., Beabout, J. W., and Jowsey, J. (1972) Femoral trabecular pattern index for evaluation of spinal osteoporosis. *Ann. Intern. Med.* **77:**63–67.

Smirnov, A. N., and Baranov, A. E. (1971) Trephine for iliac crest biopsy. *Lancet* **1:**1825–1826.

Teitelbaum, S. L., Rosenberg, E. M., Richardson, C. A., and Avioli, L. V. (1976a) Histological studies of bone from normocalcemic postmenopausal osteoporotic patients with increased circulating parathyroid hormone. *J. Clin. Endocrinol. Metab.* **42:**537–543.

Teitelbaum, S. L., Rosenberg, E. M., Bates, M., and Avioli, L. V. (1976b) The effects of phosphate and vitamin D therapy on osteopenic, hypophosphatemic osteomalacia of childhood. *Clin. Orthop.* **116:**38–47.

Thommesen, P., and Frederiksen, P. (1976) Fine needle aspiration biopsy of bone lesions: Clinical value. *Acta Orthop. Scand.* **47:**137–143.

Tonna, E. A. (1960) Osteoclasts and the aging skeleton: A cytological, cytochemical and autoradiographic study. *Anat. Rec.* **137:**251–269.

Tonna, E. A. (1965) Skeletal cell aging and its effects on the osteogenic potential. *Clin. Orthop.* **40:**57–81.

Tonna, E. A., and Cronkite, E. P. (1968) Skeletal cell labeling following continuous infusion with tritiated thymidine. *Lab. Invest.* **19:**510–515.

Villanueva, A. R. (1973) Quantitative histology of bone remodeling dynamics. *Excerpta Medica Int. Congress Series 270*, pp. 141–143.

Wakamatsu, E., and Sissons, H. A. (1969) The cancellous bone of the iliac crest. *Calcif. Tiss. Res.* **4**:147–161.

Walker, D. G. (1972) Enzymatic and electron microscopic analysis of isolated osteoclasts. *Calcif. Tiss. Res.* **9**:296–309.

Williams, J. A., and Nicholson, G. I. (1963) A modified bone-biopsy drill for outpatient use. *Lancet* **1**:1408.

Woods, C. G., Morgan, D. B., Paterson, C. R., and Gossmann, H. H. (1968) Measurement of osteoid in bone biopsy. *J. Pathol. Bacteriol.* **95**:441–447.

Yoshiki, S. (1973) A simple histological method for identification of osteoid matrix in decalcified bone. *Stain Technol.* **48**:233–238.

Young, R. W. (1962) Cell proliferation and specialization during endochondral osteogenesis in young rats. *J. Cell Biol.* **14**:357–370.

Young, R. W. (1964) Specialization of bone cells. In *Bone Biodynamics*. Edited by H. M. Frost. Little, Brown, Boston, pp. 117–139.

Appendix

Normal bone material is very hard to obtain for a number of reasons: most people die after a period of illness which almost always involves bed rest and medication. Of those who die suddenly as a result of a heart attack or trauma, a significant number have either an associated or unassociated disease such as diabetes, hypertension, or alcoholism, for which they may or may not have had treatment. Since 1963 we have collected specimens of iliac crest from individuals dying in Rochester hospitals or brought in dead as a result of an accident. The time between death and the removal and fixation of the tissue is from 2 to 24 hours, with an average interval of approximately 14 hours. In each case listed in the appendix, the cause of death and the postmortem report was available. On the basis of this report, a history of bed rest, disability, or other illness, such as rheumatoid arthritis, or any disorder commonly treated with any form of medication (e.g. epilepsy, asthma) excluded the case from the control series. Pathological findings such as a fatty liver, enlarged parathyroid, or absent ovaries also excluded the case from the normal series. The remaining cases included in the series were established to be normal and not having taken medication except for occasional mild pain-relieving drugs such as aspirin, Valium, or Darvon. The exceptions were ten cases recorded as sudden death, most of them children, who suffered acute traumatic deaths and in whom no history or pathological report was available. In some cases no cause of death is recorded; in these the bone specimen was taken, *in vivo,* during the course of an orthopaedic procedure involving an iliac crest transplant, the patient being ambulatory and having no disease or disability.

Case number[a]	Age	Sex[b]	Percentage total surface occupied by resorption	Percentage total surface occupied by formation	Mean thickness of the external and internal cortices[c]	Mean thickness of random trabeculae[d]	Video-densitometry, percentage bone per area of sample	Width of unmineralized osteoid, microns[e]	Cause of death
1	24 hrs.	F	10.4	8.1	0.6	100	80.5	5.3	Abruptio placenta in mother.
2	11 wks.	M	13.9	16.9	0.4	90	60.8	6.8	Cardiac arrest.
3	9 mos.	F	13.0	6.5	0.6	100	60.1	10.3	Sudden death.
4	11 mos.	M	12.0	8.7	0.3	100	39.6	10.8	Sudden death.
5	16 mos.	F	18.3	8.2	0.4	130	55.0	10.5	Sudden death.
6	2	M	14.1	8.6	0.5	100	41.5	10.9	Sudden death.
7	2	M	8.6	4.9	0.3	70	54.7	10.1	Pulmonary arteriosclerosis.
8	4	M	9.4	9.4	1.1	115	49.9	12.8	Car accident, DOA.
9	5	M	11.7	4.9	0.5	100	50.9	11.2	Sudden death.
10	7	M	8.3	8.7	0.8	130	50.2	—	Train accident, DOA.
11	8½	M	3.6	7.6	0.5	130	—	—	Train accident, DOA.
12	9	F	6.1	4.0	0.7	95	47.3	12.2	—
13	10	M	6.9	10.4	1.0	130	55.5	13.2	Killed in explosion.
14	10½	F	8.4	7.4	0.5	120	39.6	18.8	—
15	11	M	7.9	5.9	0.6	110	45.4	13.9	Acute trauma.
16	12	M	7.9	6.4	1.3	170	56.2	19.3	Bicycle–car accident.
17	13	M	7.6	3.2	1.4	170	61.0	16.0	—
18	13	M	8.2	10.6	1.3	140	60.4	12.5	Drowning.
19	13	M	6.2	7.4	0.9	140	59.8	14.1	Acute trauma.
20	14	M	6.8	5.6	1.6	130	53.6	—	Train accident, DOA.
21	15	M	6.1	11.4	0.8	115	59.2	16.5	Sudden death.
22	15	M	6.2	5.7	0.6	130	51.7	13.0	Car accident.
23	15	M	5.8	5.6	1.8	130	55.3	13.0	Car accident, DOA.
24	16	M	8.4	2.6	1.2	170	35.8	16.3	Motorcycle accident, DOA.

25	16	F	5.5	5.3	0.6	100	20.1	15.4	Car accident, DOA.
26	17	M	7.2	10.8	0.8	130	57.6	17.8	Car accident.
27	17	M	6.5	1.6	1.9	200	33.3	14.7	Car accident, DOA.
28	17	M	8.5	4.8	1.6	130	47.3	13.9	Suicide, gun shot.
29	18	M	6.5	2.6	1.1	130	51.0	14.9	Car accident, DOA.
30	18	M	6.3	6.9	1.5	130	47.6	14.4	Car accident.
31	18	M	4.1	4.0	1.5	125	—	14.9	Acute trauma.
32	18	M	3.3	1.3	1.9	170	65.0	13.9	Car accident.
33	18	F	4.5	2.3	1.2	130	41.2	13.4	Car accident, DOA.
34	18	F	4.8	3.6	0.9	100	48.9	13.2	Acute trauma.
35	18	F	3.9	3.9	1.1	100	48.8	15.5	Motorcycle accident.
36	18	F	3.9	6.2	1.9	130	63.2	14.7	Motorcycle accident.
37	19	M	5.4	2.3	0.6	110	49.9	13.4	Car accident.
38	19	M	3.5	5.4	1.5	130	—	16.2	Suicide, gun shot.
39	19	F	5.4	4.5	1.2	130	57.4	18.0	Car accident.
40	20	M	3.7	0.3	1.0	100	41.5	12.1	Acute trauma.
41	20	M	2.4	4.6	0.8	120	41.4	14.8	Car accident, DOA.
42	20	F	4.6	1.8	0.9	135	51.3	13.2	Car accident, DOA.
43	21	M	7.2	4.5	1.3	150	65.9	14.2	Car accident.
44	21	M	6.7	5.1	0.9	100	23.9	19.9	Car accident, DOA.
45	21	F	8.4	0.9	1.1	130	39.1	15.7	Car accident.
46	22	M	3.7	1.5	1.4	130	37.2	13.6	Car accident.
47	23	M	4.4	2.7	0.7	130	44.7	18.0	Murder, gun shot.
48	23	M	5.2	5.4	1.1	130	28.5	18.9	Drowning.
49	25	M	5.5	2.6	0.8	100	42.7	11.9	Car accident, DOA.
50	26	M	4.3	1.8	1.2	130	55.3	—	Suicide, narcotics overdose.
51	27	M	3.4	2.6	1.1	170	61.5	13.3	Car accident, DOA.
52	27	M	3.4	2.6	1.2	200	39.3	13.4	Hemorrhagic pulmonary edema.

continued

continued

Case number[a]	Age	Sex[b]	Percentage total surface occupied by resorption	Percentage total surface occupied by formation	Mean thickness of the external and internal cortices[c]	Mean thickness of random trabeculae[d]	Video-densitometry, percentage bone per area of sample	Width of unmineralized osteoid, microns[e]	Cause of death
53	27	M	2.8	2.8	1.0	130	54.8	—	Train accident, DOA.
54	28	M	6.3	0.7	0.7	200	51.7	—	—
55	28	M	3.3	2.1	0.9	130	41.4	13.0	Suicide, gun shot.
56	29	F	4.0	1.6	1.6	130	—	12.6	CO poisoning.
57	30	M	2.1	3.2	1.0	100	50.9	20.5	—
58	30	M	3.3	2.3	1.3	130	63.0	—	Electrocution.
59	30	M	2.5	1.6	0.7	170	49.0	16.8	Suicide, gunshot.
60	32	M	3.3	1.5	1.0	100	47.1	—	Suicide, gunshot.
61	32	F	3.2	2.3	1.0	130	48.6	—	Subarachnoid hemorrhage.
62	33	M	2.7	2.2	0.9	130	39.8	16.4	PO heart surgery.
63	33	F	4.3	3.0	0.8	130	56.0	14.9	Ruptured aneurysm.
64	35	M	4.8	1.9	1.8	125	39.5	12.6	Car accident.
65	37	M	4.0	1.3	1.6	130	39.8	13.7	Fall to cement, DOA.
66	37	F	2.5	3.1	1.8	140	39.0	12.3	Bus accident.
67	38	M	3.2	3.4	0.7	130	37.4	15.5	Cerebral aneurysm.
68	39	M	1.6	3.8	1.1	150	—	—	—
69	41	M	4.3	2.9	1.5	130	57.3	20.2	CO poisoning, DOA.
70	41	M	4.8	1.6	0.8	130	26.0	—	Head injury.
71	41	F	4.5	0.6	1.2	100	48.2	—	Subarachnoid hemorrhage.
72	41	F	4.0	0.6	0.9	130	46.3	15.1	Suicide.
73	42	F	4.1	0.4	1.6	130	42.2	—	—
74	43	M	2.9	2.4	1.0	130	42.4	13.2	Acute MI.
75	43	M	3.9	1.5	1.0	130	53.2	13.8	—
76	44	M	3.2	0.8	0.8	130	27.5	14.8	Subarachnoid hemorrhage.

77	45	M	6.8	2.2	2.0	150	31.2	14.8	Car accident.
78	45	M	3.6	2.4	0.7	100	24.3	16.2	Suicide, gunshot.
79	45	F	1.7	3.6	0.6	110	47.0	15.3	Car accident, DOA.
80	46	M	4.0	3.9	1.0	120	25.8	18.9	Car accident, DOA.
81	47	M	2.4	0.8	1.1	130	22.0	19.1	Acute coronary insufficiency.
82	48	M	5.4	0.9	0.8	100	33.7	—	MI.
83	48	F	3.8	4.3	1.0	100	49.7	18.3	—
84	49	M	3.7	2.0	0.8	130	30.0	13.4	Suicide by hanging.
85	49	M	4.5	0.7	1.3	130	29.8	15.9	Acute coronary occlusion.
86	50	M	4.4	1.9	0.8	200	38.7	17.2	Electrocution.
87	51	M	2.8	3.0	2.1	120	36.0	13.9	Sudden death.
88	51	M	4.1	1.2	0.7	160	40.7	18.3	CVA.
89	51	F	5.7	1.6	0.9	100	36.2	15.3	MI.
90	53	M	4.5	1.8	1.0	150	28.8	15.7	Suicide, gunshot.
91	54	M	4.6	1.8	2.1	190	31.6	14.9	Cornchopper accident.
92	55	M	3.1	0.9	0.6	175	25.1	13.6	Coronary insufficiency.
93	55	M	6.9	1.0	1.5	190	42.7	10.7	Coronary insufficiency.
94	55	M	4.7	4.0	1.0	240	36.5	14.9	Sudden death.
95	55	M	2.3	1.3	1.0	130	34.2	—	CO poisoning.
96	55	F	3.3	0.9	0.5	100	47.9	11.2	PO heart surgery.
97	56	M	2.3	2.3	1.8	100	55.7	11.9	CVA.
98	57	M	3.6	4.6	1.2	130	59.8	14.6	MI.
99	57	M	1.1	3.3	0.9	120	48.5	17.4	Car accident, DOA.
100	58	F	1.7	1.3	1.1	130	34.8	10.5	Ruptured aneurysm.
101	59	M	5.1	1.8	0.6	130	40.5	11.2	Coronary insufficiency.
102	59	F	3.3	3.1	0.8	130	47.5	18.5	Acute MI.
103	60	M	3.3	1.1	0.6	100	22.9	—	—
104	60	M	4.9	1.8	0.6	100	31.4	16.2	Suicide by hanging.
105	60	F	3.1	1.9	0.9	150	47.4	14.2	—

—continued

continued

Case number[a]	Age	Sex[b]	Percentage total surface occupied by resorption	Percentage total surface occupied by formation	Mean thickness of the external and internal cortices[c]	Mean thickness of random trabeculae[d]	Video-densitometry, percentage bone per area of sample	Width of unmineralized osteoid, microns[e]	Cause of death
106	60	F	5.0	0.2	1.4	150	45.5	QNS	MI.
107	60	F	4.4	6.7	1.1	100	44.5	14.3	Sedative overdose
108	61	M	1.2	4.0	1.0	130	34.4	14.9	Accidental strangulation.
109	62	M	2.8	3.0	0.6	100	44.6	14.6	—
110	62	F	3.0	2.4	0.8	100	36.8	18.1	Subarachnoid hemorrhage.
111	63	F	4.1	1.1	0.8	170	19.3	QNS	Sudden death.
112	64	M	5.2	0.2	0.4	170	33.8	19.8	Ruptured aortic aneurysm.
113	64	M	3.5	1.3	0.8	150	—	—	Multiple injuries, 20 ft fall
114	64	F	4.5	3.1	0.6	170	36.2	12.6	—
115	64	F	3.2	2.6	0.8	70	40.5	15.5	Ruptured carotid aneurysm.
116	65	M	6.3	1.5	0.5	130	47.3	15.1	Cerebral hemorrhage.
117	66	F	3.1	2.1	1.3	130	28.0	14.4	Car accident.
118	67	M	4.7	0.4	0.5	130	29.5	QNS	Ruptured aortic aneurysm.
119	67	M	4.4	2.9	1.3	170	48.7	15.7	PO aneurysm repair.
120	68	M	2.2	1.3	1.0	130	42.0	14.6	MI.
121	68	M	3.3	1.1	0.7	130	31.2	QNS	Acute coronary insufficiency.
122	68	F	5.5	5.1	0.5	105	33.6	—	Car accident.
123	69	F	6.4	0.4	0.5	80	30.9	—	Cardiac infarction.
124	70	M	4.0	0.5	1.1	130	50.1	16.5	Car accident.
125	70	F	3.2	1.3	0.3	100	36.1	—	—
126	70	F	3.4	2.2	0.4	80	40.5	14.8	Car accident.
127	71	M	6.6	2.4	0.4	90	34.3	14.9	Coronary insufficiency.
128	71	M	4.9	0.8	0.6	130	33.0	—	MI.

129	72	M	6.0	2.2	1.0	160	50.9	16.1	Coronary insufficiency.
130	72	M	3.1	0.4	0.8	100	44.1	QNS	Coronary insufficiency.
131	72	M	3.2	2.1	1.3	170	50.1	QNS	GI hemorrhage.
132	73	M	5.5	2.7	0.5	110	26.6	18.0	Ruptured aneurysm, aorta.
133	73	F	5.3	0.5	1.3	120	42.0	QNS	Coronary insufficiency.
134	74	F	2.3	4.6	0.8	130	—	—	—
135	75	M	4.4	1.2	1.0	100	42.8	17.3	Coronary insufficiency.
136	76	M	3.6	0.9	—	150	—	12.9	Cerebral infarction.
137	76	F	6.4	1.6	1.1	150	57.1	QNS	Cardio respiratory arrest.
138	76	F	5.5	2.6	0.5	140	24.7	—	Homicide by strangulation.
139	76	F	3.1	1.9	1.1	120	37.6	QNS	Sudden death.
140	76	F	—	0.9	0.5	110	30.1	12.3	Cerebral hemorrhage.
141	77	F	4.9	3.4	0.4	70	29.2	—	—
142	78	F	2.5	3.0	0.5	140	42.8	14.7	MI.
143	78	F	3.5	0.8	0.6	110	36.6	14.1	Subarachnoid hemorrhage.
144	80	F	4.4	6.5	1.0	130	59.0	12.8	Coronary insufficiency.
145	81	F	5.0	0.4	0.7	100	35.3	QNS	—
146	82	F	2.9	4.9	0.8	170	—	—	Ruptured liver.
147	84	F	2.5	1.2	1.2	110	37.2	13.6	MI.
148	85	M	3.8	1.5	1.0	100	30.9	—	—
149	85	M	5.1	0.8	0.6	110	24.2	—	Pedestrian struck by car.
150	85	F	3.8	2.4	0.5	170	24.4	14.2	Cerebral hemorrhage.
151	88	M	3.8	0.9	0.7	100	33.3	—	—
152	88	M	2.6	1.5	0.4	110	30.8	13.6	Head injury.
153	89	M	3.0	2.1	0.9	100	49.5	12.2	Acute MI.

a Consecutive with age.
b F=Female, M=male.
c Mean of 6 measurements.
d Mean of 20-30 measurements.
e Mean of 12 measurements.

Index

157